THE NEUROLOGICAL TREATMENT FOR NEARSIGHTEDNESS AND RELATED VISION PROBLEMS

A Guide to Vision Improvement
Based on 30 Years of Research

THE NEUROLOGICAL TREATMENT FOR NEARSIGHTEDNESS AND RELATED VISION PROBLEMS

A Guide to Vision Improvement Based on 30 Years of Research

John William Yee

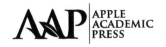

Apple Academic Press Inc.
3333 Mistwell Crescent
Oakville, ON L6L 0A2
Canada USA

Apple Academic Press Inc.
1265 Goldenrod Circle NE
Palm Bay, Florida 32905
USA

© 2020 by Apple Academic Press, Inc.

First issued in paperback 2021

Exclusive worldwide distribution by CRC Press, a member of Taylor & Francis Group

No claim to original U.S. Government works

ISBN 13: 978-1-77463-417-2 (pbk)
ISBN 13: 978-1-77188-732-8 (hbk)

CIP data on file with Canada Library and Archives

Library of Congress Cataloging-in-Publication Data

Names: Yee, John William, author.
Title: The neurological treatment for nearsightedness and related vision problems : a guide to vision improvement based on 30 years of research / John William Yee.
Description: Toronto ; New Jersey : Apple Academic Press, 2020. | Includes bibliographical references and index.
Identifiers: LCCN 2019018631 (print) | LCCN 2019019016 (ebook) | ISBN 9780429465048 (ebook) | ISBN 9781771887328 (hardcover : alk. paper)
Subjects: | MESH: Refractive Errors--therapy | Myopia--therapy
Classification: LCC RE925 (ebook) | LCC RE925 (print) | NLM WW 300 | DDC 617.7/55--dc23
LC record available at https://lccn.loc.gov/2019018631

Apple Academic Press also publishes its books in a variety of electronic formats. Some content that appears in print may not be available in electronic format. For information about Apple Academic Press products, visit our website at **www.appleacademicpress.com** and the CRC Press website at **www.crcpress.com**

DEDICATION

To the late William Yee, who always knew that
it was possible.

CONTENTS

ABBREVIATIONS

ADD	addition
AOA	American Optometric Association
BTI	brain trauma injury
K reading	keratometer reading
OD	oculus dexter (right eye)
ortho K	orthokeratology
OS	oculus sinister (left eye)
OU	oculus uterque (both eyes)
PD	pupil distance
PMMA	polymethyl methacrylate
RGP	rigid gas permeable
Rx	prescription
V/A	visual acuity

FOREWORD

He has given me a great gift. A dangerous gift. The gift of knowing.

—Dr. Bennet Omalu, from the movie Concussion.

I have 30 years' experience in the study of nearsightedness prevention. John William Yee has made a major personal effort to design preventive methods for this difficult problem, and these methods are effective.

It is always difficult to pioneer an alternative treatment in a field as conservative as optometry, and it takes a bold "soul" to take these first steps. John has made a strong personal commitment to his research. He offered his findings internationally. His participants were from different countries around the world, and they have attested to the effectiveness of his system. The originality of John's work is very important, but of far greater importance is the humanitarian aspect of that work—that he continues to support certain individuals who cannot afford good vision at no cost to them.

In this book, he, in turn, offers this knowledge to professionals. Progress in this field will also require professionals to provide personal sacrifice of themselves and their time to help others. His pioneering development of "Ortho C" shows promise to effectively prevent nearsightedness at the threshold. His standard of professionalism and his commitment to support the welfare of others sets a high example for all of us.

—**Otis S. Brown**
Author of *How to Avoid Nearsightedness,*
Waynesboro, PA, United States

PREFACE

It's unbelievable how much you don't know about the game you've been playing all your life.

—Mickey Mantle

PRIMARY REFRACTIVE ERRORS

I invented something I want to share with you: the multiplier effect (Yee, 2012). I designed it to treat primary refractive errors. A primary refractive error refers to mild and moderate nearsightedness with similar prescriptions in both eyes or with a disparity of less than −0.50 D. Mild nearsightedness is from −0.25 D to −0.75 D and moderate nearsightedness is from −1.00 D to −1.75 D.

THE MYOPIC MODEL

The mild and moderate myopic eye represents the myopic model. It represents how the eye became nearsighted on its own accord. There are less extraneous variables affecting the eye in those ranges. The higher ranges of nearsightedness are susceptible to more variables offsetting the expected outcome after applying ortho C. The eye can become progressively worse due to something else outside the myopic model, and those variables have to be dealt with first.

TREATING REFRACTIVE ERRORS SLIGHTLY OUTSIDE THE MYOPIC MODEL

I am also providing information on how to deal with primary refractive errors where both eyes are slightly outside the model. Such an eye offers a partial resistance. (Refer to the chapters *The Procedure* and *The Theory Behind the Resistance Tests* for more information.)

SECONDARY REFRACTIVE ERRORS

I also invented something else: the indirect effect (2012). I designed it to treat secondary refractive errors, such as: anisometropia, anisometropic amblyopia, and compound astigmatism where the astigmatism is high. To minimize the resistance from anisometropia, one eye should be in the mild or moderate myopic range, and both eyes are within the myopic model. The eye is correctable as long as one eye is within the mild or moderate range. It does not matter if the other eye is outside that range. To minimize the resistance from high astigmatism, the myopic portion should be mild or moderate. The eye may not be totally correctable in the short term, but there would be a significant reduction in refractive error. For example, I had a participant with the following prescription −1.50–1.25 × 180 who wears just a −0.50 D glasses after performing the Modified Preliminary Drill a few times.

THE APPLICATION OF NEUROLOGY

The treatment relies mainly on neurology (on resetting the correct neuro-muscular message) and less on physiotherapy (such as applying relaxation exercises and massaging the eye). You initially became nearsighted when the incorrect neuromotor message was relayed to the intraocular and extraocular muscles. It is the incorrect message that locks the lens and the eyeball in their myopic shape. The tension of the oblique muscles initiated the incorrect message. When the eye became myopic, the regulatory role changes from the ciliary muscle to the oblique muscles.

The extra tension of the extraocular muscles does not induce spasticity. Instead, it neurologically imposes a ceiling on how much the ciliary muscle can relax to allow the lens to flatten to make out something clearly far away. The ciliary muscle of a mild or moderate myopic eye can still bulge some more for near focusing, and it can still flatten out to a certain extent from its bulged shape for distant focusing (up to the ceiling imposed). The lens in its open neutral shape is different from its occluded neutral shape. The rectus muscles do not lose their tensile strength when the tension of the extraocular muscle elongates the eye slightly. The rectus muscles can still retract the eyeball upon releasing the tension of the oblique muscle. (Refer to the chapter *How It Reverses Nearsightedness* for more information on the reversal process.)

The correct neurological message depends on the function of vision, and vision is a cognitive process. If a myopee had both eyes occluded, the "contact lens draw" would not work. If the Standard Drill was performed with the eyes opened, however, the reversal process would take about 5 min—to insert the lenses, perform the drill, and take them out. The ortho C lens acts as a catalyst to activate the ciliary muscle and the rectus muscles. It is the motor cortex that relays the proper message to those muscles to synchronize the lens and eyeball once the oblique muscles are "loosened" by a "contact lens draw." If the mild and moderately myopic eye is within the myopic model, the outcome from ortho C is almost identical to laser surgery in clarity and retention.

It took me over 30 years to perfect the methodology, or at least as close to perfection as I could come, before I opened a research facility to gather more data. I was lucky to have participants all over the world helping me with the research. Some continued to correspond with me to supply long-term data.

GRANTING YOU THE RIGHTS

I am granting to you the rights to apply ortho C to improve the vision of anyone who approaches you with the intention of correcting their myopia by ortho C. Mild and moderate myopia are easier to treat compared to the other ranges. All you have to do is follow the step-by-step instructions for the specific drill outlined in the chapter *What to Do*. The chapter *The Procedure* provides the context surrounding the drill such as designing the lens, determining the sequence of wear, and conducting resistance tests.

I wrote the book for a professional audience. By professional, I am referring to the medical profession, naturopath, neurologists, psychiatrist, psychologist, and researchers—as well as the eye care specialist. I strove for clarity in my writing for the benefit of other disciplines. In some chapters you are also an imaginary patient so that you can visualize certain hypothetical situations. I hope that by sharing my discovery with you in the following pages, it can generate interdisciplinary insights for further research.

VISION STATEMENT

I never did intended to monopolize my findings and then charge a ridiculous price for the treatment; but I did want to patent it to prevent others from doing just that. I abide by the philosophy of the Canadian inventor Frederick Grant Banting who discovered insulin. Any invention that proposes a cure should be affordable, it should be available to everyone, it should not be inferior, and it should not be monopolized by a corporation.

INTRODUCTION

If something is important enough, you should try even if the possible outcome is failure.

—Elon Musk

I opened a research facility with the help from some of my students. I wanted to gather more data from participants interested in my proposed treatment for nearsightedness. I was warned by my peers that I would fail. Seeking participants from a broader population meant that I would incur more extraneous variables—or variables that can offset the expected outcome. Some of them may take the following form: different ocular problems in addition to myopia (such as astigmatism and loss of depth perception), different degrees of myopia, different kinds of myopia (such as anisometropia and progressive myopia), and different ways one can become myopic (in terms of what the participant did, genetic factors, etc.). But I had an idea how to control them.

I received no grants, no funding…nothing. I managed somehow to break even over the last 9 years. Most of my participants insisted on giving me something to cover my cost so that I can stay in business, and my intern students always wanted to help by suggesting new ideas and new products to deal with the business side of the operation. There were certain periods, however, when failure seemed to be the likely outcome.

I later realized that my research was not restricted by the boundary of my city or even by the border of my country. Most of the participants were from other countries, such as the United States, United Kingdom, Australia, France, Germany, Russia, Hong Kong, Hungary, Italy, Mexico, the Netherlands, Malaysia, Romania, South Africa, and countries I never heard of. I learned from them as much as they learned from me.

WHAT I FOUND

I found that if mild or moderate myopia was within a certain range, it is possible to stimulate it in such a way that it would immediately develop the natural tendency to revert back to its premyopic shape. The treatment relies on a plain "flexible" pair of contact lenses (without any prescription). Perhaps a good name for the procedure is orthoculogy, which is Latin for correcting the whole eye, or "ortho C" for short. It influences both the crystalline lens and the eyeball to become less myopic instead of just the lens. (Most researches attempt to reverse nearsightedness by manipulating just the lens. Refer to the chapter *What Natural Relaxation Drills Can and Cannot Do* for more information.)

The average initial improvement is two or three lines on the Snellen chart—regardless that it is more difficult to gain two lines in the lower half of the chart than the upper half. The results are quicker than laser surgery, and there are no side effects or discomfort requiring recovery. The *speed* of the improvement suggests that there is a neurological component. By reinstating the correct neurological message, the eye tends to revert back to its premyopic shape. The *degree* of improvement presupposes that mild and moderate myopia eye tends to fall within the myopic model. Usually, the patient is not exposed to certain extraneous variables in that range. The *retention* of the improved visual acuity suggests that the eyeball also participated in the reversal process. Otherwise, the crystalline lens would do all the work. If the lens had to compensate for the myopic shape of the eyeball as well as its own myopic shape, certain condition would create an excessive "effort to see." By expending 100% effort or more instead of 50%, there is the risk of inducing asthenopia. (Refer to the chapters *The Effort to See* and *Letting Go* for more information.)

An ortho C lens improves your vision naturally in the sense that it is a neurological process. There are no implants involved, such as implanting a "ring" onto your cornea (cornea ring implant), or implanting a lens between your natural lens and the iris (intraocular lens implant), or implanting another cornea onto your existing cornea. There are no "retainer" lenses to wear once your vision improves—as in the case of orthokeratology, or "ortho K" for short, which is Latin for "correcting the cornea."

Do not confuse ortho C with ortho K. Ortho K attempts to correct your refractive error by flattening the cornea with a very flat contact lens instead of attending to the myopic shape of the crystalline lens or the eyeball. Ortho C does not flatten the curvature of the cornea. Its curvature does not change, and this can be verified by taking another K reading (or keratometer reading) after your vision improves. The treatment depends on a "contact lens draw." If the cornea had altered, it would interfere with the "draw." Ortho C would not work properly. (Refer to the chapter *Reinstating the Correct Message* for more information.)

A BRIEF OVERIEW

A brief overview on the treatment is given in the section *What to Do*. It outlines the drills the patient needs to do in relation to the type of myopia—mild or moderate myopia with no disparity between each eye, anisometropia, compound astigmatism, etc. The chapter *The Procedure* outlines the context behind the specific drill: designing the lens, ordering the lenses, and what to do with them once you receive them from the lab, etc.

THE LAYOUT OF THE BOOK

PART 1

The first part of the book is on the etiology of myopia. Knowing the cause of myopia will help you realize why I intend to treat it in a certain way and why the design of an ortho C lens needs to follow certain specifications. You have to know the problem before you can treat it. The main culprit is the excess tension of the oblique muscles. (Refer to the chapter *The Main Culprit* for more information.)

My hypothesis on near-point stress can be demonstrated first by treating the myopic eye, then inducing a relapse, and then applying the same treatment again. I would first treat the eye by ortho C—by relaxing the part of the myopic eye affected by near-point stress: the oblique muscles. It suggests that the relaxation of those muscles by a "contact lens draw" contributes to emmetropia. The outcome is the opposite of near-point stress. It is possible to induce a relapse by simulating a condition that resembles near-point stress. It indicates that the excess tension of the oblique muscles is a contributing factor. It is also possible to reverse the myopia again by ortho C. It indicates that a "contact lens draw" produces an alternative outcome by "loosening" the oblique muscles.

Of course I did not encourage any participant to engage in such an experiment. It was conducted accidently on several occasions. After "reducing" the higher ranges of myopia by orthoculogy (as opposed to "correcting" mild or moderate myopia), some clients accidently induced a relapse by wearing their replacement glasses all the time instead of just relying on them mainly for the distance. Although the glasses were under-corrected for the distance to allow them to see 20/25 or 20/30 (depending on their visual requirements), it was still overcorrected in the near and intermediate range.

PART 2

The second part of the book is on the treatment. The treatment is based on targeting the main culprit: the excessive tension of the oblique muscles. The reversal process takes only minutes after applying the multiplier effect or the indirect effect or both. It suggests that there is a neurological component (as mentioned in the chapter *Neurological Implications*). The increase in retention compared to the other drills to treat a primary refrac-tive error indicates that the sclera as well as the crystalline lens participated in the correction. The main reason why I restricted my research to the mild and moderate myopic range is that there are less extraneous variables interfering with the expected outcome. Mild and moderate myopia tends to fall within the myopic model and have a low resistance (to ortho C). The myopic model represents how nearsightedness sets in uninterrupted.

I also included a treatment for secondary refractive errors that are within the myopic model: astigmatism, anisometropia, and anisometropic amblyopia in addition to mild and moderate myopia. High astigmatism, or a significant distortion of the cornea or lens, can be treated if the myopic portion of the eye is mild or moderate. Anisometropia, which is a differ-ence in prescription between the right and left eye, can also be effectively treated if one eye is in the mild or moderate range while the other eye is in the midrange.

I also included a treatment for primary refractive errors that are slightly outside the myopic model and offer a partial resistance. There are resistance tests designed to test for the possibility of a partial resistance. The tests are not just test per se. They are like mini drills that set up different conditions to activate an eye with a partial resistance. Once you know which resistance test stimulates an improvement in visual acuity, you will know which drill to apply. For example, if the Fourth Resistance Test activated an eye with a partial resistance, then you know you have to assign the Modified Standard Drill. (Refer to the chapter *The Theory Behind the Resistance Tests* for more information.)

In relation to a specific refractive error, the theories and their applications are found in the following chapters:

The theory behind the treatment for mild and moderate myopia with no disparity in prescription between each eye, for example, is given in the chapter *The Theory Behind the Standard Drill*. Its application in the treatment for that refractive error is given in the chapter *Treating Mild and Moderate Myopia*. The theory behind the treatment for anisometropia, for example, is given in the chapters *The Theory Behind the Preliminary Drill* and *The Theory Behind the Modified Preliminary Drill*. Their application in the treatment for that refractive error is given in the chapter *Treating Anisometropia*. The theory behind the treatment for astigmatism, for example, is given in the chapter *The Theory Behind the Modified Preliminary Drill*. Its application in the treatment for that refractive error is given in the chapter *Treating Astigmatism*.

PART 3

The third part of the book is on verification. When I submitted rough copies of the manuscript to some of my colleagues for their input (before I wrote the section on *Verification*), they would frequently say, "But can you prove it?"

They alluded not so much to the etiology of nearsightedness and the effectiveness of ortho C in dealing with it as proposed in the chapter *Near-Point Stress*. Instead of a correlational relationship, it seems the scientific community is more interested in the reliability of the methodology itself: the efficiency of the apparatus (the contact lenses), the methods applied (the different drills), and the theories arrived at. In that respect, the verification consists of demonstrating the reliability of the methodology as expressed in the chapters: *Reinstating the Correct Message, Follow-ups, Troubleshooting*, and *Case Examples*.

I attempt to demonstrate the reliability of the methodology as follows:

- By emphasizing the importance in adhering to specifications, it demonstrates that the contact lens corrects only the part or parts of the eye that deviated and only within the range of deviation.

- By outlining what to look for in a follow-up, it demonstrates the importance of adhering to protocol. Adhering to protocol reinforce the reliability of the drills.
- By citing actual troubleshooting approaches to demonstrate the reliability of the standard method of treatment and the design of the lens.
- By providing case examples that relied on a pretest posttest design to exemplify standardization.

WHAT TO DO

For we live by faith, not by sight.

—2 Corinthians 5:7

I am giving you the main drills to deal with your patient's type of refractive error. It takes about 5 min to perform the drill. From the pretest and posttest results, you can determine the improvement in visual acuity. Refer to the chapter *Wearing Schedule* for information on maintaining the improvement and extending the retention period. The process is not that difficult. I included some actual cases in the chapter *Case Examples*. Also refer to *The Procedure* for the context surrounding the drills.

THE STANDARD DRILL

I designed the Standard Drill to treat myopia from −0.75 D to −1.75 D with the same prescription for both eyes or with a disparity of no more than −0.25 D between each eye. It offers the longest retention period before you have to perform the drill again for maintenance due to the multiplier effect. The Standard Drill consists of the following supplementary drills: The Distance Drill and the Snellen Chart Drill. The following are some highlights to keep in mind. Both the right and left lenses are worn together in Steps 1 and 2. The patient performs the Distance Drill with the better eye first in Step 1 while covering the other eye and then with the weaker eye next in Step 2 while also covering the other eye. The lens for the better eye must be worn separately first in Step 3 and then the lens for the weaker eye next in Step 4 while performing the Snellen Chart Drill. In Step 5, the patient performs the Distance Drill again with no lenses on. (Refer to *The Procedure* for the preparation leading to the application of the drill and to *The Theory Behind the Standard Drill* for more information.)

THE PRELIMINARY DRILL

I designed the Preliminary Drill to treat anisometropia. The patient usually applies it prior to the Modified Preliminary Drill to relax the ciliary muscle. The patient may also apply it prior to the Standard Drill in order to adapt to the lenses. The Preliminary Drill consists of the following supplementary drills: The Distance Drill and the Snellen Chart Drill.

The following are some highlights to keep in mind. The right and left lenses are worn separately in all the steps of the drill. Each lens is worn alternatingly. The patient wears the lens in the weaker eye first in Step 1. Then he takes the lens off. Then he wears the lens in the better eye next in Step 2. Then he takes the lens off, etc. It establishes the wearing sequence in the other steps: the weaker eye first and then the better eye. (Refer to *The Procedure* for the preparation leading to the application of the drill and to *The Theory Behind the Preliminary Drill* for more information.)

MODIFIED PRELIMINARY DRILL

Another important drill is the Modified Preliminary Drill. I have applied it to treat different types of refractive errors: simple astigmatism, myopia plus high astigmatism, anisometropia plus astigmatism, and anisometropia combined with anisometropic amblyopia plus astigmatism. The Modified Preliminary Drill consists of the following supplementary drills: The Distance Drill and the Snellen Chart Drill.

The following are some highlights to keep in mind. The right and left lenses are worn separately in all the steps of the drill. Each lens is worn "inline." The patient wears the lens in the weaker eye first in Steps 1 and 2. Then he takes the lens off. Then he wears the lens in the better eye next in Step 3 and 4. Then he takes the lens off.

The exception to the regular wearing sequence is in the treatment for compound anisometropia and anisometropic amblyopia. The patient wears the lens in the better eye first in Steps 1 and 2 and in the weaker eye in Steps 3 and 4. He wears the lens for only 15 s when performing the Distance Drill in Steps 1 and 3 when treating anisometropia. It is more sensitive than myopia. (Refer to *The Procedure* for the preparation leading to the application of the drill and to *The Theory Behind the Modified Preliminary Drill* for more information.)

THE STANDARD DRILL TO TREAT MILD AND MODERATE MYOPIA FROM −0.75 D TO −1.75 D

1. Wear both lenses. Look outside at an object about 500 or 1000 ft away with the *better eye.* (Look 500 ft away if you have moderate myopia. Look 1000 ft away if you have mild myopia.) **Cover** the other eye. Hold the palm 2–3 in. from the eye to prevent instrument myopia. Keep both eyes open. Do the Distance Drill for 30 s.

2. With both lenses still on, look at an object about 500 or 1000 ft away with the *weaker eye.* **Cover** the other eye. Look at the same object in Step 1. Hold the palm 2–3 in. from the eye. Keep both eyes open. Do the Distance Drill for 30 s. Then take off the lens on the weaker eye.

3. With only the lens on the *better eye,* perform the Snellen Chart Drill. **Cover** the other eye. Hold the palm 2–3 in. from the eye. Keep both eyes open. Stand 5.0 ft away from the chart. Read line 7 five times at a rate of 1 s per letter. Then take the lens off.

4. Insert the lens on the *weaker eye* and perform the Snellen Chart Drill. **Cover** the other eye. Hold the palm 2–3 in. from the eye. Keep both eyes open. Stand 5.0 ft away from the chart. Read line 7 five times at a rate of 1 s per letter. Then take the lens off.

5. *Without* any lenses on, look outside at an object about 500 or 1000 ft away with *both* eyes. Look at the same object in Step 1. Do the Distance Drill for 1 min with both eyes. *Not* with each eye separately.

THE PRELIMINARY DRILL TO TREAT ANISOMETROPIA

1. Wear the lens on the *weaker eye* only. Look outside at an object about 500 ft away. **Do not cover** the other eye. Keep both eyes open. Do the Distance Drill for 15 s. Then take the lens off.

2. Wear the lens on the *better eye* only. Look outside at an object about 500 ft away. **Do not cover** the other eye. Look at the same object in Step 1. Keep both eyes open. Do the Distance Drill for 15 s. Then take the lens off.

3. Wear the lens on the *weaker eye* only. Perform the Snellen Chart Drill with the *weaker eye* first. **Cover** the other eye. Hold the palm about 2–3 in. from the eye. Keep both eyes open. Stand 5.0 ft

away from the chart. Read line 7 five times at a rate of 1 s per letter. Then take the lens off.

4. Wear the lens on the *better eye* only. Perform the Snellen Chart Drill with the *better eye*. **Cover** the other eye. Hold the palm about 2–3 in. from the eye. Keep both eyes open. Stand 5.0 ft away from the chart. Read line 7 five times at a rate of 1 s per letter. Then take the lens off.

5. Without any lens on, look outside at an object about 500 ft away with the *weaker eye*. **Cover** the other eye. Look at the same object in Step 1. Leave a slight gap 2–3 in. from the eye. Keep both eyes open. Do the Distance Drill for 30 s.

6. Without any lens on, look outside at an object about 500 ft away with the *better eye*. **Cover** the other eye. Look at the same object in Step 1. Leave a slight gap 2–3 in. from the eye. Keep both eyes open. Do the Distance Drill for 30 s.

THE MODIFIED PRELIMINARY DRILL TO TREAT SIMPLE ASTIGMATISM, MILD MYOPIA, OR COMPOUND MYOPIA AND HIGH ASTIGMATISM

1. Wear the lens on the *weaker eye* only. Look outside at an object about 500 ft away. **Do not cover** the other eye that does not have the lens on. Keep both eyes open. Do the Distance Drill for 30 s.

2. With the lens still on the *weaker eye*, perform the Snellen Chart Drill. **Cover** the other eye. Hold the palm 2–3 in. from the eye. Keep both eyes open. Stand 5.0 ft away from the chart. Read line 7 five times at a rate of 1 s per letter. Then remove the lens.

3. Wear the lens on the *better eye* only. Look at an object about 500 ft away. ***Do not cover*** the other eye. Look at the same object in Step 1. Keep both eyes open. Do the Distance Drill for 30 s.

4. With the lens still on the *better eye*, perform the Snellen Chart Drill. **Cover** the other eye. Hold the palm 2–3 in. from the eye. Keep both eyes open. Stand 5.0 ft away from the chart. Read line 7 five times at a rate of 1 s per letter. Then remove the lens.

5. Without any lens on, look outside at an object about 500 ft away with the *weaker eye*. **Cover** the other eye. Look at the same object in Step 1. Leave a slight gap 2–3 in. from the eye. Keep both eyes open. Do the Distance Drill for 30 s.

6. Without any lens on, look outside at an object about 500 ft away with the *better eye*. **Cover** the other eye. Look at the same object in Step 1. Leave a slight gap 2–3 in. from the eye. Keep both eyes open. Do the Distance Drill for 30 s.

THE MODIFIED PRELIMINARY DRILL TO TREAT ANISOMETROPIA OR COMPOUND ANISOMETROPIA AND HIGH ASTIGMATISM

1. Wear the lens on the *weaker eye* only. Look outside at an object about 500 ft away. **Do not cover** the other eye that does not have the lens on. Keep both eyes open. Do the Distance Drill for 15 s.
2. With the lens still on the *weaker eye*, perform the Snellen Chart Drill. **Cover** the other eye. Hold the palm 2–3 in. from the eye. Keep both eyes open. Stand 5.0 ft away from the chart. Read line 7 five times at a rate of 1 s per letter. Then remove the lens.
3. Wear the lens on the *better eye* only. Look at an object about 500 ft away. **Do not cover** the other eye. Look at the same object in Step 1. Keep both eyes open. Do the Distance Drill for 15 s.
4. With the lens still on the *better eye*, perform the Snellen Chart Drill. **Cover** the other eye. Hold the palm 2–3 in. from the eye. Keep both eyes open. Stand 5.0 ft away from the chart. Read line 7 five times at a rate of 1 s per letter. Then remove the lens.

THE MODIFIED PRELIMINARY DRILL TO TREAT COMPOUND ANISOMETROPIA AND ANISOMETROPIC AMBLYOPIA

1. Wear the lens on the *better eye* only. Look outside at an object about 500 ft away. **Do not cover** the other eye that does not have the lens on. Keep both eyes open. Do the Distance Drill for 15 s.
2. With the lens still on the *better eye*, perform the Snellen Chart Drill. **Cover** the other eye. Hold the palm 2–3 in. from the eye. Keep both eyes open. Stand 5.0 ft away from the chart. Read line 7 five times at a rate of 1 s per letter. Then remove the lens.
3. Wear the lens on the *weaker eye* only. Look at an object about 500 ft away. **Do not cover** the other eye. Look at the same object in Step 1. Keep both eyes open. Do the Distance Drill for 15 s.

4. With the lens still on the *weaker eye*, perform the Snellen Chart Drill. **Cover** the other eye. Hold the palm 2–3 in. from the eye. Keep both eyes open. Stand 5.0 ft away from the chart. Read line 7 five times at a rate of 1 s per letter. Then remove the lens.

THE SUPPLEMENTARY DRILLS

The following are instructions for the supplementary drills within the above drills:

DISTANCE DRILL

With the ortho C lens on, direct your attention to an object approximately 500 or 1000 ft away depending on the specific drill. Perform the Distance Drill for the duration specified in the recommended drill. Then take the lens out immediately before ortho K sets in.

You can scan the house across the street, the cars, or the trees. Rather than staring at the whole object, scan the particular parts of the object. Trace the outline of each particular object with your nose. Pretend that it is a very sharp pencil. Trace, for example, the outline of the wheels of the car, the windshield, the frame, etc.

Then zoom in on something else if there is another object at that distance and trace it the same way. Do not trace anything closer or farther away. If there is not another object, then keep tracing the outline of the different parts of the present object.

Do not try to blot everything up in your visual field. When you are scanning the branches of a tree, for example, trace the branches, the trunk, the leaves, etc. Do not try to blot up the whole tree without scanning it. And do not scan too fast. You want the image to come into focus.

SNELLEN CHART DRILL

You would stand 5.0 ft away from the Snellen chart. It has to be exactly 5.0 ft away. Each incremental distance influences the targeted muscles differently—even if the difference is just half a foot away. When you read line 7, read from letter to letter at a rate of 1 s per letter. Do not read too fast. Wait for the letter to come into focus before you move on to the next letter. If the letters do not come into focus, blink a few times to nudge the ciliary muscle to relax. Do not squint to force the letter into focus. If you cannot see line 7, try reading line 6 instead. Avoid straining the eye to see the letters.

Read the chart in artificial light. Hang the chart up in an area where the lighting is consistent. Its brightness should not change each time you do the exercise. Do not read it under natural light (light from outside). It is more challenging to read it in artificial light. The same chart is used to check your vision. When you are testing your vision, a similar chart should be by a natural source of light because it allows you to see subtle differences much easier.

ADDITIONAL INSTRUCTIONS

TAKE THE LENS OUT IMMEDIATELY

When you are about to take the lens out, do not waste time looking at something close for an extended period, do not answer the phone, do not be distracted by the TV, etc. Do not forget that the treatment is mainly neurological. Take the lens out immediately to avoid the chance that the wrong neuromotor message might be sent in response to some activity that is not related to the drill.

MINIMIZE THE MOVEMENT OF THE LENS

To minimize the movement of the lens, hold the upper lid up and anchoring it against the upper eye socket. You want the upper lid to clear the lens because a tight lid may interfere with the "contact lens draw." It is common for the upper lid to attach to the upper part of the contact lens when wearing a conventional RGP lens. If you blink without holding the upper lid up, the upper lid will knock the lens down during the downward movement, and it will draw it up during the upward movement before the lens centers again. (The lens must move because it is sitting on a layer of liquid. It does not touch the cornea.) These extra movements will cut into the time the lens stimulates the eye. You can still blink, but try to minimize it. When you do blink occasionally when the upper lid is held up, only the lower lid will come into contact with the lens—which causes less disturbance. You still want to control the blink by attempting not to blink as often.

Sometimes a hard blink can pop the lens out. The lens is slightly flatter than the cornea. If you blink hard, the lid may wedge between the lens and the cornea. During the initial stage, it is a good idea to hold one hand under the eye in case it pops out. It is natural for the eye to try to reject the lens before it adapts to it.

NOT TO BE DONE AT NIGHT

Never do the drill at night. A "focal point draw" will not be activated. Also do not do the drill on an overcast day. The "focal point draw" will not be as efficiently. Perform the drill on a slightly cloudy day is best. Try to avoid a very sunny day. A clear day is OK.

STAY INSIDE

Do not go outside while performing the Distant Drill. The aperture of the eye will become smaller, and it can interfere with a "focal point draw." The image will be clearer not because of a "focal point draw." The aperture becomes smaller due to the brightness, and the decrease in the size of the pupil contributes to the clarity of the object. The muscles will not be doing as much work. Stay inside the residence and look out. Step a few feet away from the window sill. When you are inside, the aperture is wider. It requires the muscles to do some work in bringing an image into focus.

MEASURING THE DISTANCE FOR THE DISTANCE DRILL

You can estimate the suggested distance for the Distance Drill. The best way to measure 500 ft away, for example, is to take 250 paces. Measure the distance of your step first from toe to toe with a ruler. Try to maintain that width as you laid out 250 paces. The object does not have to be exactly 500 ft away. Come as close to it as possible. The longest hallway inside a mall where my clinic is located is 300 ft. My participants still get good results when performing the Distance Drill.

PART 1
Defining the Problem

CHAPTER 1

WHY ORTHO C?

ABSTRACT

You have to know the problem before you can treat it. The onset of myopia indicates that there is a change in the regulatory role on how the eye brings an object into focus. A common cause is near-point stress, and it forces the crystalline lens to bulge. I want to take it a step further and explain how it entices the eyeball to become myopic. The oblique muscles tend to tighten up to alleviate the tension of the ciliary muscle. Once those muscles maintain the excessive tension, the elongated eyeball becomes fixed. It sets the stage for the theory behind the treatment. You have to reverse how the eye became myopic due to near-point stress. A "contact lens draw" decreases the tension of the oblique muscles to allow a "focal point draw" to take place concurrently before the myopic shape of the lens and eyeball can retract neurologically for distant focusing.

What makes ortho C so special? For one thing, if your refractive error is within the myopic model, the treatment only takes about 5 min: the time it takes to insert the lens, perform the drill, and take the lens out. It produces a noticeable difference within that time—especially if you have a primary refractive error. It is quicker than laser surgery, and it is not necessary to set aside time to recover from any incisions. It suggests that ortho C involves a neurological process. (Refer to the chapter *Neurological Implications*.) The following are highlights of the problem and proposed treatment.

1.1 THE PROBLEM

1.1.1 NEAR-POINT STRESS

During my research, I explored the cause of myopia first before proposing a treatment. I based the treatment on its etiology. If I just relied on the symptoms in terms of the different types and degrees of nearsightedness, there would have been a lot of guesswork. The cause of nearsightedness is outlined in the chapters *Near-point Stress* and *The Main Culprit.*

To alleviate the tension of the ciliary muscle due to near-point stress, the oblique muscles would tighten up. The intention is to elongate the eyeball to bring the retina closer to the focal point of a very close object (which is behind the retina). By maintaining the excessive tension of the oblique muscles over a period of time, it activates an improper neurological response. A revised neurological message influences the ciliary muscle to tighten up continuously. The lens assumes a bulged shape for all ocular ranges. Another neurological message influences the rectus muscles to relax to allow the eyeball to elongate. These relationships of the myopic eye are established by the common cranial nerve 3 (or C3).

1.1.2   THE HYPOTHESIS ON THE PROBLEM

The motor cortex regards the myopic eye to be in near focus mode due to the excessive tightness of the oblique muscles. It maintains the myopic shape of the crystalline lens and eyeball even when the eye attempts to make out an object far away. (Refer to the chapter *The Main Culprit* for the context surrounding the hypothesis.)

1.1.3   MYOPIC MODEL

The myopic model represents an eye that became nearsighted naturally (on its own accord). Ortho C assumes that your patient's nearsightedness falls within the myopic model. It presupposes that the excess tension of the oblique muscles indirectly sets the tension of the ciliary muscle due to near-point stress. There is no mechanical connection between the crystalline lens and the oblique muscles. The tension of the oblique muscles imposes a ceiling on how much the lens can flatten out. In the meantime, the lens can still bulge (for near work) or flatten out up to the restriction imposed by the oblique muscles (for distant work). Thus, the ciliary muscle is still flexible. Spasticity had not set in. (Refer to the chapter *The Main Culprit* for more information.)

Mild and moderate myopia exemplifies the myopic model. There are less extraneous variables interfering with the expected outcome. The midrange and severe myopic eye tends to fall outside the model. Those ranges are susceptible to more extraneous variables and are more difficult to treat.

1.1.4   THE THEORIES ON THE PROBLEM

The myopic model introduces the following theories behind the problem (Refer to the chapter *Neurological Implications* for more information):

The first theory on the relationship between the oblique muscles and the ciliary muscle of the myopic eye can be expressed as follows: the excessive tension of the oblique muscles causes the ciliary muscle to become tense to entice the crystalline lens to bulge. The first part of the Preliminary Drill presupposes that such a condition exists. It targets the thickness of the ciliary muscle in the treatment of anisometropia. The drill produces a direct and indirect effect to the extent that it would increase the relaxation of the ciliary muscle without flattening the eyeball by the same proportion. By not flattening the lens' occluded neutral shape, it does not stimulate the eyeball to retract prematurely. The application of the drill to treat anisometropia would not work if the first myopic relationship did not exist. (Refer to the section on *The Treatment* in this chapter for more information on the indirect effect.)

The second theory on the relationship between the oblique muscles and the rectus muscles of the myopic eye can be stated as follows: the excessive tension of the oblique muscle causes the rectus muscles to relax to allow the eyeball to elongate. The direct and indirect effects in the first and second part of the Modified Preliminary Drill presuppose that such a condition exists. The drill would not work if the second myopic relation-ship did not exist. (Refer to the section on *The Treatment* in this chapter for more information on the direct and indirect effect.)

The third theory on the synchronization of the two dual relationships of the myopic eye can be expressed as follows: the tendency for the crystalline lens to bulge also causes the eye to elongate. The first part of the Standard Drill exemplifies that such a condition exists. The multiplier effect needs to flatten the occluded neutral shape of the crystalline lens before the eye can retract. The drill would not work if the third myopic relationship did not exist. (Refer to the section on *The Treatment* in this chapter for more information on the multiplier effect.)

1.1.5 DEALING WITH THE ROOT OF THE PROBLEM

The treatment deals with the root of the problem instead of just treating the symptom. The chapter *The Main Culprit* identifies the main problem that maintains your nearsightedness: the excessive tension of the oblique muscles. By loosening those muscles with an ortho C lens, it triggers the correct neuromuscular message to address all parts of the eye affected by myopia. The treatment becomes more complete.

1.2 THE TREATMENT

1.2.1 THE HYPOTHESIS ON THE TREATMENT

The hypothesis in reference to the proposed treatment is the reverse of the hypothesis of how the eye became myopic. When a "contact lens draw" is combined with a "focal point draw," it triggers a reversal in myopia by "loosening" the oblique muscles. When the shapes of the lens and eyeball are not restricted by the tension of the oblique muscles, the brain considers the eye to be emmetropic. It stimulates the eye neurologically to correct itself. The process is the reverse of near-point stress. (Refer to the chapter *Designing the Lens* for the context surrounding the hypothesis.)

1.2.2 THE THEORY ON THE TREATMENT

Prior to ortho C, the motor cortex ignores the myopee's perception of a distant object even though the subject knows that it is far away. Due to the tension of the oblique muscles, the brain interprets the eye to be in near focus mode. It bypasses the neurosensory message of a blur distant object. When a "contact lens draw" combines with a "focal point draw," it expands the vertical height and horizontal width of the eye (when viewing the eye from the front). It "loosens" the oblique muscles' grip around the eyeball. The motor cortex will then take the subject's depth perception of a distant image into account. It recognizes that the eye is in distant focus mode. It reinstates the correct neuromuscular message to allow distant objects to come into focus. (Refer to the chapter *How It Reverses Nearsightedness*.)

1.2.3   THE MULTIPLIER EFFECT

I designed the Standard Drill to treat a primary refractive error. It represents the application of the multiplier effect (Yee, 2011). It starts with a direct effect—the effect of the contact lens on the eye wearing the lens. It takes place when a change in the crystalline lens' occluded neutral shape triggers the eyeball to change. It is the opposite of near-point stress. The lens' occluded neutral myopic shape needs to change first before the eyeball can change. It reverses the two dual relation-ships between the oblique muscles and ciliary muscle and the oblique muscles and the rectus muscles due to the common cranial nerve 3. (Refer to the chapter *How It Reverses Nearsightedness* for the design of the ortho C lens and to chapters *The Theory Behind the Standard Drill* and *Treating Mild and Moderate Myopia* for an elaboration of the multiplier effect.)

The lens' occluded neutral shape is different from its open neutral shape. The focal point of the former is farther from the retina after blocking the other eye during the drill. When it moves closer to the retina after the lens flattens, there is still a sufficient gap to allow the eyeball to retract. The focal point of the latter is closer to the retina when opening both eyes during the drill. The crystalline lens already took on a flatter shape prior to performing the drill. When it flattens some more after the drill, the focal point is on the retina. Only the lens shifted. There is no room for the myopic eyeball to follow suit.

(For more information on the lens' occluded neutral shape refer to the chapters *What Natural Relaxation Drills Can and Cannot Do, The Theory Behind the Resistance Tests,* and *The Theory Behind the Standard Drill.*)

The multiplier effect takes place when the direct effect on the eye wearing the lens is transmitted to the eye not wearing the lens—the occluded eye. The indirect effect on the occluded eye is amplified by the contact lens on that eye to create a multiplier effect (on the occluded eye). The multiplier effect is transmitted back to the open eye to reinforce the direct effect (on the open eye). It contributes to the increase in visual acuity and retention. The eyeball (or sclera) tends to reduce its elongation. It all takes place in Step 1 in the first part of the drill. The second part of the drill shortens the elongation of the sclera further.

1.2.4   THE INDIRECT EFFECT

The indirect effect, or indirect influence as I sometimes called it, can also create a partial multiplier effect (Yee, 2011). The multiplier effect can be thought of as a series of indirect effects, but it was designed to treat a primary refractive error where the prescription of each eye is the same or with a disparity of −0.25 D. I had to come up with something less intense to treat secondary refractive errors. I apply the indirect effect in the treatment for anisometropia, anisometropia and anisometropic amblyopia, anisometropia and high astigmatism, and myopia and high astigmatism. A multiplier effect would not work on those types of refractive errors.

The Modified Preliminary Drill produces a series of indirect effects. It starts with the direct effect. It takes place when the crystalline lens' open neutral shape flattens partially in Step 1. Holding that partial change, the eyeball is stimulated to change in Step 2. The eyeball "shifts" because the partial flattening of the lens allowed some room to retract. There is an adequate gap between the focal point and the retina. The eyeball reduces its elongation to correct the residual myopia. Again, the process is the opposite of near-point stress.

An indirect effect takes place when the direct effect is transmitted to the other eye not wearing the lens. The indirect effect is not amplified since the other eye does not have a contact lens on. The message is not relayed back to the eye originating it (as in the multiplier effect). The indirect effect would reinforce the direct effect on that eye once it wears a contact lens in Steps 3 and 4. (Refer to the chapter *The Theory Behind the Modified Preliminary Drill* for more information.)

1.2.5   A NATURAL TREATMENT

Ortho C is a natural treatment even though it relies on a contact lens. It is possible to reset the correct neurological message by relaxing the oblique muscles. The deviated shapes of the crystalline lens and eyeball tend to revert back to their original shape naturally. You do not have to physically force the crystalline lens or the eyeball to assume a certain shape. It is actually the motor cortex that relaxes, stretches, and strengthens different muscles to coax the cornea, lens, and eyeball back to their premyopic shape once ortho C reinstates the proper neurological message. For example, the contact lens does not differentiate between anisometropia and astigmatism. The drill to treat both refractive errors is the same: the Modified Preliminary Drill. The brain fine tunes the treatment. The "contact lens draw" "loosens" the oblique muscles to initiate it. The simulation from an ortho C lens on the eye is the opposite of the effect of a minus lens. The "contact lens draw" induces a progressive improvement as opposed to progressive myopia.

1.2.6 THE MYOPIC EYE'S RESISTANCE

Initially I only intended to correct the low resistance eye—or an eye that offers a low resistance against the treatment. Now I can extend the treatment to include the partial resistance eye—or an eye that offers a partial resistance against the treatment. If an eye offers a partial resistance, it does not necessarily mean that the improvement will be partial. The deviation can still be within the myopic model. The outcome after treating anisometropia, for example, is similar to the outcome after treating mild and moderate myopia with no disparity in prescription between the right and left eye. On the other hand, ortho C can still attend to an eye outside the myopic model with a partial resistance. A resistance test determines the extent of the resistance. (Refer to the chapter *The Theory Behind the Resistance Tests*.)

1.2.7 THE RESISTANCE TESTS

How fast and how much improvement you can expect depends on the resistance of the eye. It is determined by conducting a series of resistance tests as outlined in the chapter *The Procedure* and *The Theory Behind the Resistance Tests*. The myopic eye can exhibit a low resistance, a partial resistance, or a high resistance. The resistance tests provide useful information on the flexibility of the ciliary muscle. It can be flexible or inflexible. If it is inflexible, it may have incurred a partial spasm or a total spasm. You can refer to the resistance tests as a flow chart to help you identify the type of resistance.

1.2.8 UNLOCKING THE TENSION OF THE CILIARY MUSCLE

The theory behind these tests is that it is not just a resistance test. The eyeball cannot correct itself unless the ciliary muscle is flexible enough to activate the lens to change. The resistance that holds the lens in a myopic shape must be unlocked first. The resistance tests are not just tests per se but are also possibilities for unlocking the partial spasm incurred by the ciliary muscle. Once it is unlocked, it provides a hint of the eye's resistance level.

If the mild or moderate eye with a primary refractive error is within the myopic model, there should be a low resistance. There is a reduction in exposure to extraneous variables in that range. The First Resistance Test should unlock the tension of the ciliary muscle.

If the mild or moderate eye with a primary refractive error is slightly outside the myopic model, its partial resistance would have a different response. The gain in visual acuity is lower. Its depth perception is also lower. (Refer to the chapter *The Theory Behind the Resistance Tests* for more information.)

1.2.9   WEARING SCHEDULE

To maintain the improvement and to address progressive myopia, the patient would wear the lenses regularly and perform the drill—again for about 5 min. (The chapter *Treating Progressive Myopia* emphasizes that you should adhere to a wearing schedule to address progressive myopia as well as myopia.) Initially, the patient would perform the drill two or three times a week for 2 weeks and then determine the retention period afterwards at different intervals. (Refer to the chapter *Wearing Schedule* for more information.)

1.2.10   IMPORTANT RULES

It is important to adhere to the following rules:

- Wear the lenses for therapeutic purposes only—not as a visual aid.
- Apply a drop of solution onto the lens before insertion.
- Do not experiment with the ortho C lens.

The patient cannot wear the lens too long. Ortho C involves mainly neurology, not physiotherapy. Once you reset the neurological message, it is not necessary to continue resetting it after your vision improves. For example, if you are treating mild myopia, the eye can regain its normal shape after one application. If the patient continues to wear the lens throughout the day instead of taking them out, the improved visual acuity would deteriorate.

You can only reverse the deviated shape of the eye. You cannot alter the part of the eye that has not deviated or alter it beyond its deviation. Once the lens gains its normal shape for distant focusing, you cannot try to force it to change some more. It can be demonstrated by inserting an ortho C lens on your normal eye—assuming your visual acuity is 20/20. Your vision would become blurred. You cannot reset the vision of an eye that does not need to be reset.

Remind the patient to apply a drop of solution onto the lens before insertion. Otherwise a "contact lens draw" may not work properly. The "contact lens draw" has to be all around the perimeter of the lens. A drop of solution onto the contact lens prior to insertion smooths out the imperfections of the cornea surface to permit an even "draw." (Refer to the chapter *How it Reverses Nearsightedness* and to the *Addendum* on inserting an ortho C lens for more information.)

Also remind the patient not to conduct any experiments with the ortho C lens. Again, the treatment involves neurology and not just physiology. Extraneous variables can be induced by experimenting just for the sake of conducting an experiment.

KEYWORDS

- myopia
- neurology
- near-point stress
- etiology
- motor cortex
- regulatory role
- myopic model

CHAPTER 2

THE PARTS OF THE EYE AFFECTED

ABSTRACT

The base curve of an ortho C lens is flatter than the curvature of the cornea by an amount expressed in diopters. It is equal to the total deviation of the myopic eye also measured in diopters. The assumption behind ortho K is that the curvature of the cornea would flatten by that amount before an object in the distance can come into focus, but ortho C is different from ortho K. An interesting phenomenon behind ortho C is that the improvement in vision is not due to a flatter cornea. It is an indication that the treatment involves resetting the correct neurological message to alter the curvature of the lens and eyeball. The design of an ortho C lens is almost the same as an ortho K lens. The main difference is in the thickness. To appreciate how altering just the thickness can correct a primary refractive error, the chapter examines the parts of the myopic eye that can deviate from the emmetropic eye.

2.1   THE SHAPE OF THE CRYSTALLINE LENS

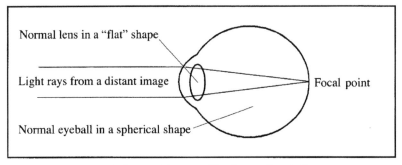

FIGURE 2.1   The normal shape of the crystalline lens and eyeball.

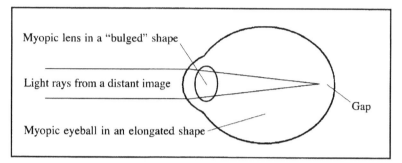

FIGURE 2.2   The myopic shape of the crystalline lens and eyeball.

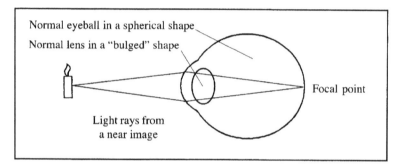

FIGURE 2.3   The normal shape of the crystalline lens for near focusing.

The crystalline lens of a normal or emmetropic eye assumes a flat shape when it focuses on a distant object as illustrated in Figure 2.1. It flattens out when the center of the lens becomes shorter from front to back. The lens changes to a bulged shape when it focuses on a near object as illustrated in Figure 2.3. It bulges when the center of the lens becomes longer from front to back.

The lens of a mild or moderate myopic eye, on the other hand, cannot flatten out sufficiently when it attempts to make something out far away as shown in Figure 2.2. It bulges or assumes a round shape instead. It should only bulge when it focuses on something close-up as shown in Figure 2.3—not on something far away.

2.2   THE SHAPE OF THE EYEBALL

A spherical eyeball in its normal shape is illustrated in Figure 2.1. The myopic eyeball, however, is in an elongated shape. When the myopic eye attempts to bring a distant object into focus, the focal point falls short of the retina as shown in Figure 2.2. The image then appears blur. It is not just due to the elongated shape of the eye, but also to the bulged shape of the lens. Mild ranges of myopia are mainly attributed to the bulged shape of the crystalline lens; but moderate, midrange, and severe ranges of myopia are attributed to both the myopic shape of the crystalline lens and eyeball.

When I make reference to the eyeball, I am actually referring to the sclera. Only the outermost part of the myopic eyeball "shifted" or became elongated. The innermost part is attached to the optic nerve. Although the optic nerve do offer some slack, it is the sclera which defines the shape of the eyeball (Grierson, 2000).

The application of ortho C to treat mild and moderate myopia takes into account how much the crystalline lens and eyeball became myopic. When treating mild myopia, most or all of the deviation is due to the lens. When treating moderate myopia, most of the deviation is still inherited by the lens, and the eyeball is slightly more myopic compared to mild myopia but not as myopic compared to midrange or severe myopia.

2.3   THE SHAPE OF THE CORNEA

The cornea is the transparent membrane at the front part of the eye which protrudes from the sclera. It has a "steeper" curvature compared to the eyeball. If the cornea takes on an irregular shape due to the misalignment of the rectus muscles, it can interfere with your vision (Yee, 2012). This condition is known as astigmatism—or more specifically, corneal astigmatism.

If you have simple corneal astigmatism or astigmatism that exists by itself, it is due to the irregular shape of the cornea. The deviated shape of the cornea will not be immediately corrected. In the short term, the correction involves the crystalline lens adjusting its shape to compensate for the distortion. In the long term, there may also be a reduction in the deviated shape of the cornea as the "contact lens draw" continues to stimulate the rectus muscles to align (Yee, 2012).

If you have simple lenticular astigmatism, it is due to the irregular shape of the crystalline lens. It is dealt with in the same way as reducing the myopic shape of the lens. The crystalline lens itself would change immediately. No other parts of the eye would have to compensate for the irregular shape of the lens (Yee, 2013a).

2.4   THE SHAPE OF THE CRYSTALLINE LENS, EYEBALL, AND CORNEA

When astigmatism combines with the myopic shape of the lens and eyeball, it is referred to as compound astigmatism. If the patient's astigmatism is 1.00 D or less, depending on the "sphere", the brain can usually compensate for it. If it is more than −1.00 D, it will affect your vision; but ortho C can attend to it at the same time as your myopia. (Refer to the *Specifications* for the amount of flatness to account for astigmatism.)

There are also other types of refractive errors that can combine with myopia such as presbyopia (erroneously called old age vision) and anisometropia (the difference in the prescription of each eye). The assumption in this book is that your presbyopia in compound presbyopia (or presbyopia combined with myopia) is less than your myopia. If presbyopia is your primary problem, I will discuss its treatment in a separate publication. The treatment is different. Anisometropia will be discussed in this book.

2.5   ADDRESSING THE MYOPIC SHAPES OF THE LENS AND EYEBALL

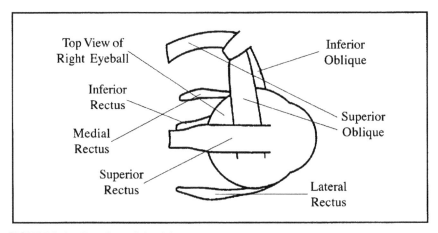

FIGURE 2.4   Top view of the right eye.

To reverse how the eye became myopic, you need to attend to the culprit that maintains the shape of the myopic lens and eyeball: the tension of the oblique muscles. The oblique muscles are the pair of extraocular muscles attached to the top and bottom of the eye at right angle to the rectus muscles as illustrated in Figure 2.4. Their primary function is to rotate the eyeball, and their secondary function is turning it.

The tension of the oblique muscles neurologically maintains the myopic shape of the crystalline lens as well as the eyeball. When the eye became myopic, it created two dual relationships that did not exist before in the emmetropic eye: the relation between the oblique muscles and ciliary muscle and the relation between the oblique muscles and the rectus muscles. (Refer to the chapter *Neurological Implications* for more information.)

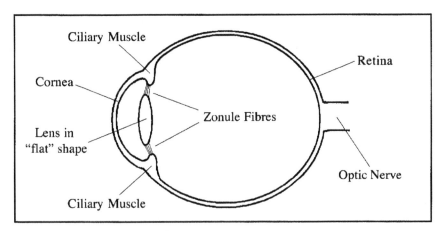

FIGURE 2.5   Cross-section of the eye.

The ciliary muscle is a ring circling the lens. It is attached to the crystalline lens by zonule fibers. Refer to the cross sectional diagram in Figure 2.5. It controls the shape of the crystalline lens. When the ciliary muscle relaxes, it recedes. The fibers become taut and pull on the lens to flatten it for distant focusing. When the muscle becomes tense, it thickens. It is like how your biceps expand when you flex them. The fibers become loose. The slack allows the lens to assume its normal round shape for near focusing. When myopia sets in, the ciliary muscle responds to the excessive tension of the oblique muscles by also becoming tense to entice the lens to bulge.

The rectus muscles are the four extraocular muscles that run lengthwise across the eye. There is a rectus muscle on each side of the eye and on the top and bottom of the eye as illustrated in Figure 2.4. Their primary function is turning the eye, and their secondary function is rotating it. When myopia sets in, the rectus muscles respond to the excessive tension of the oblique muscles by relaxing to entice the eyeball to elongate.

2.6   THE EFFECT OF ORTHO C

Once ortho C "loosens" the oblique muscles, the motor cortex responds to the neurosensory message by sending a revised neuromuscular message. It creates a series of physiological changes. It reverses what took place when the eye became myopic. It relaxes the ciliary muscle and increases the tautness of the rectus muscles. It alters the structure of the myopic eye for distant focusing by enabling the crystalline lens to flatten out from its bulged shape (after relaxing the ciliary muscle) and the eyeball to retract from its elongated shape (after increasing the tension of the rectus muscles).

KEYWORDS

- emmetropic
- astigmatism
- corneal astigmatism
- lenticular astigmatism
- base curve
- flatter curve
- steeper curve

CHAPTER 3

NEAR-POINT STRESS

ABSTRACT

Light rays are divergent when an object is up close. The crystalline lens becomes round to bring it into focus. When looking at an object less than 16 in. away, the lens bulges to its maximum. By maintaining that shape for an extended period, the "effort to see" becomes excessive. The eyeball would elongate to alleviate some of the stress placed on the ciliary muscle. The drawback with bringing the retina closer to the focal point (by elongating the sclera) rather than the focal point closer to the retina (by enticing the lens to bulge) is that the oblique muscles may not return to their relaxed state under normal conditions. The excessive tension of the oblique muscles produces a different neurological message for distant focusing. It is as if though you are still engaged in near focusing even when looking far away.

"Why am I nearsighted?" your clients may ask if they were told by their eye care specialists that they need glasses to make out objects far away. They may not get a definite answer—even if they searched online. There is a lack of a definitive theory. It is possible that there are several causes. The model that I am proposing attempts to address the question before seeking a treatment.

3.1 THE EMMETROPIC EYE

How the emmetropic or normal eye brings an object into focus is based on the theory of Helmholtz. It stipulates that only the crystalline lens performs that task, and the ciliary muscle regulates the lens. A near image comes into focus when the ciliary muscle becomes tense to enable the crystalline lens to bulge. An image far away comes into focus when the ciliary muscle relaxes to allow the crystalline lens to flatten out (Caban, 1993).

The theory of Helmholtz refers to the emmetropic eye. You need a different model to explain the onset of myopia. Before the eye became myopic, most likely the theory of Helmholtz still applies. The ciliary muscle determines the shape of the crystalline lens. The lens changes readily from a bulged shape to a flat shape in response to the need for an immediate change in focus from near to far and vice versa. The myopic eye, however, relies on different muscles to regulate the lens and eyeball. The following question was never critically examined: "How did the eye became elongated if the muscles controlling it did not participate in focusing prior to the onset of myopia?"

3.2 EXCESSIVE CLOSE WORK

One theory to explain the disruption in how the eye normally functions is the engagement in excessive close-up work, or what is commonly called "near-point stress." The literature explores the concept in terms of a change in the shape of the lens. I will take it a step further and explain how the eyeball fits into the picture and how the myopic shape of the lens and eyeball became fixed.

3.2.1 AFFECTING THE CRYSTALLINE LENS

During close work, the focal point is behind the retina due to the divergent rays of light from a near object as opposed to parallel rays when an object is far away. The crystalline lens cannot remain in its neutral flat shape but would have to become round or assume a bulged shape. The increase in the steepness of the lens converges the rays to bring the focal point back onto the retina.

The ciliary muscle would have to tighten up. The flexing of the muscle makes it larger in the same way as how your biceps enlarges when you flex it. The reduction in the space between the lens and the ciliary muscle as a result allows the zonule fibers to become slack to allow the lens to bulge. Once the lens reaches its maximum bulged shape, the "effort to see" would become excessive if the focus was maintained in the near range, especially closer than 16 in., for an extended period (Yee, 2013b).

3.2.2 AFFECTING THE EYEBALL

The eyeball would start to elongate to alleviate some of the stress placed on the ciliary muscle. The tension of the oblique muscles increases to force the eyeball to assume an elongated shape. The rectus muscles would respond by becoming less taut. Instead of the lens bulging beyond the maximum to bring the focal point onto the retina, the eyeball elongates to bring the retina closer to the focal point to reduce some of the effort associated with extensive near focusing (Yee, 2013b).

The drawback with bringing the retina closer to the focal point in this manner is that the oblique muscles may not return to their relaxed state under normal conditions. In turn, it would lock in the myopic shape of the crystalline lens and eyeball. Ghosh et al. (2014) found that the axial length of the eye increased during near work. They concluded that ciliary muscle tension and extraocular forces were contributing factors. It was consistent with Muftuoglu et al.'s (2009) findings of thicker ciliary muscles in eyes with high axial lengths due to myopia.

The phenomenon is commonly experienced by students. After engaging in prolong near work, the blackboard can appear blur for a few seconds. Extensive reading without taking a break is not the only condition that can trigger near-point stress. After playing video games for a long time, objects in the distance can appear blurred momentarily. Besides children during development, anyone can experience it. If you acquired the habit of constantly texting on the cell phone or looking at the text on the computer screen for hours without taking a break, it tends to produce the same effect.

3.3 A DIFFERENT NEUROLOGICAL MESSAGE

If the excessive tension of the oblique muscles during extensive near focusing becomes permanent, it invokes a different neurological message for bringing a distant object into focus. The brain interprets the excess tension as an eye that is in near focus mode. It is as if though you are still engaged in near focusing even when you are looking far away. The new neuromuscular message locks in the myopic shape of the lens and eyeball.

The oblique muscles act as a relay switch to send the new message to the ciliary muscle (to cause the lens to bulge) as well as to the rectus muscles (to cause the eyeball to elongate). There is no physical link between the oblique muscles and the ciliary muscle, but the oblique muscles can still influence the ciliary muscle to tighten up to allow the lens to bulge; and there is no physical link between the oblique muscles and the rectus muscles, but the oblique muscles can still influence the rectus muscles to relax to allow the eyeball to elongate. These relationships of the myopic eye are established by the common cranial nerve—cranial nerve 3 (or C3).

The myopic model lays the groundwork for the theories on first myopic relationship (between the ciliary muscle and the oblique muscles), the second myopic relationship (between the rectus muscles and the oblique muscles), and the third myopic relationship (between the crystalline lens and the sclera). The theories on these relationships are discussed in the chapter *Neurological Implications*.

3.4   DEMONSTRATING NEAR-POINT STRESS

3.4.1   INDUCING A RELAPSE

The negative impact from near-point stress can be demonstrated by the following experiment. First, I would treat the myopic eye with an ortho C lens. It relaxes the oblique muscles. The participant would usually see an improvement in visual acuity after the first application. After a day or two, I would induce a relapse by subjecting the eye to a condition that represents near-point stress. It would tighten the oblique muscles and trigger a relapse. Then afterwards I would treat the eye by ortho C again. Most likely, it would reverse the decline in visual acuity if the participant did not engage in near-point stress for an extended period. By applying the same method to improve the myopia prior to the relapse, it presupposes that a "contact lens draw" reversed the induction of near-point stress.

Of course I did not encourage any participant to engage in such an experiment, but it was often conducted accidently. After "reducing" the higher ranges of myopia by orthoculogy (as opposed to "correcting" mild or moderate myopia), some clients accidently induced a relapse by wearing their replacement glasses all the time instead of just relying on them mainly for the distance. Although the new prescription was weaker (undercorrected for the distance to allow them to see 20/25 or 20/30 depending on their visual requirements), it was still overcorrected in the near range. The "effort to see" was high because the focal point was projected farther behind the retina by the minus lens. The eye immediately reverted back to its former myopic shape when an incorrect neurological message overrides the correct message for distant focusing. The process was the reverse of how I corrected their myopia.

3.4.2   REVERSING THE RELAPSE

The participants accidentally induced a relapse by engaging in a negative condition that resembles the condition prior to ortho C. It induces near-point stress because a minus lens causes the divergent rays from a near object to diverge even more. The focal point is farther behind the retina. The extra effort required to close the gap to bring an object into focus produced a relapse. The crystalline lens needs to assume a bulged shape before that could take place.

If I applied ortho C again to reverse the relapse to a state that resembles the participant's condition prior to the relapse, then ortho C negatively correlates with near-point stress. I would go along with the contention that it is still a correlational relationship instead of a causal relationship. The contention is that the induction of a relapse by wearing a minus lens may not quite resemble near-point stress. It may involve other variables, but I still think it is an accurate representation of near-point stress since the demonstration can be duplicated. The answer to "Why am I nearsighted?" involves an interdisciplinary explanation: biological, behavioral, and neurological.

3.5   DISCUSSION

3.5.1   MYOPIA DUE TO A NEUROLOGICAL INTERPRETATION

The nearsighted eye is actually an eye that is stuck in near focus mode. The interpretation that the eye is in near focus mode due to the neurosensory message from the tightness of the oblique muscles takes precedence over the perception of a distant image via the visual cortex. Although you know that the object is far away, the motor cortex responds by sending a revised neuromotor message to carry out the function of near focusing. The degree of revision depends on the tension of the oblique muscles (Yee, 2011).

3.5.2   REINFORCING THE THEORY OF HELMHOLTZ

When an ortho C lens reverses the refractive error by relaxing the oblique muscles, I am not replacing Helmholtz's theory. Ortho C stimulates the myopic eye to reverse its curvature in an attempt to restore emmetropia. It is not enhancing the vision of the normal eye.

If you do not need glasses, and you still insist on "high definition vision" by means of ortho C, your visual acuity would actually deteriorate. You would be treating something that does not need treatment. By attempting to change how the existing visual system operates instead of reinstating it, ortho C can conflict with the emmetropic state of the eye.

The eye naturally strives to achieve emmetropia during development and postdevelopment. An ortho C lens can disturb the relationship between the crystalline lens and the eyeball in the same way as how a minus lens can disrupt that relationship (as discussed in more detail in the chapter *Treating Progressive Myopia*). So, ortho C may actually reinforce the theory of Helmholtz.

KEYWORDS

- Helmholtz
- emmetropia
- near-point stress
- divergent rays
- zonule fiber
- axial length
- cranial nerve
- visual cortex

CHAPTER 4

THE MAIN CULPRIT

ABSTRACT

When an eye became myopic, the regulatory role switches from the ciliary muscle to the oblique muscles. The change is neurological rather than mechanical. If it was mechanical, the elongation of the eye causes the zonule fibers to become slack when the vertical distance across the middle of the eye decreases after the eyeball elongates. The lens would bulge independent of the ciliary muscle. In the myopic eye, however, the ciliary muscle becomes thicker (due to an increase in tension) before the lens bulges. If the lens bulges due to the elongation of the eyeball, then the ciliary muscle does not need to tighten up (or become thicker); but since the ciliary muscle of a myopic eye is thicker, it suggests that the lens bulges first before the eye elongates—not the other way around. The myopic model provides important information in the theory behind the treatment of myopia. The myopic lens must flatten first before the myopic eyeball can retract.

4.1 CHANGE IN REGULATORY ROLE

If you explain how the eye functions in terms of how the ciliary muscle changes the crystalline lens' curvature to bring objects at different distances into focus, you are explaining the regulatory role of the emmetropic eye. With the myopic eye, there is the question, what causes the eye to maintain its myopic shape? How does that affect the regulatory role of the emmetropic eye?

When an eye became myopic, the impact from near-point stress offers a hint that the regulatory role switched from the ciliary muscle to the oblique muscles. The common cranial nerve C3 (cranial nerve 3) is the neurological pathway that allows the oblique muscles to relay a message to the ciliary and rectus muscles. Once the brain picks up the neurosensory message (the excess tension of the oblique muscles), a neuromotor message is sent to the ciliary muscle via cranial nerve 3 to engage the lens in near focus mode. It takes precedence for both near and distant focusing. The same message is simultaneously relayed to the rectus muscles also via cranial nerve 3. The rectus muscles would relax accordingly to allow the eyeball to elongate if necessary (Yee, 2011).

There are other models which also make reference to the extraocular muscles' participation in defining the shape of the eye in near focus mode. According to Doonan (1984), for example, the oblique muscles tighten up and the rectus muscles also ease their tension. The difference between Doonan's model and the myopic model is that the myopic model refers to the myopic eye while Doonan's model refers to the emmetropic eye. Another difference is that according to Doonan's model, the rectus muscles take on a regulatory role. According to the myopic model, the regulatory role of the oblique muscles takes over when the eye becomes myopic; and before the eye became myopic, the theory of Helmholtz still applies.

But let us consider Doonan's model in reference to the myopic eye. The intention is not to highlight the shortcoming of that model. The author applied the model to the emmetropic eye. I am merely borrowing the concept to shed some light on the comparison between a mechanical and a neurological regulatory role in the myopic eye.

4.2   MECHANICAL REGULATION

If the rectus muscles, instead of the oblique muscles, play a dominant role in regulating the shape of the myopic eye, it implies that the eyeball and the crystalline lens became myopic at the same time. Under this mechanical relationship, the lens would not have deviated unless the eyeball had deviated. It means that near-point stress involves both the lens and eyeball. The lens would not independently influence the eye to elongate. The deviation would be shared between the crystalline lens and eyeball—as explained below in the section *A Restriction on the Lens*. However, there are mild and moderate cases where the crystalline lens deviated more than the eyeball.

4.3   NEUROLOGICAL REGULATION

Instead of the rectus muscles assuming a regulatory role, it is possible that the oblique muscles neurologically take on that role. Once the spasm of the oblique muscles sets in, the brain regards the eye to be in near focus mode even when you are looking far away. The oblique muscles act as a relay switch to channel the modified neuromuscular message to the ciliary and rectus muscles to orchestrate the change in distant focusing (Yee, 2011).

4.4   AN IMPORTANT DIFFERENCE

An important characteristic that differentiates the neurological aspects of the myopic model from the mechanical aspects is the regulatory role between the oblique muscles and the ciliary muscle (and thus the lens). There is no mechanical connection between the crystalline lens and the oblique muscles, but those muscles can still impose a restriction on how much the lens can flatten. (I would later refer to this as the first myopic relationship in the chapter *Neurological Implications.*)

The change in regulatory role is tied in to near-point stress. The eyeball became elongated when the crystalline lens cannot bulge any further. The regulatory role transfers over to the oblique muscles. It provides an important piece of the puzzle in understanding how an eye becomes nearsighted and why ortho C can treat it so quickly. The ability for ortho C to treat the mild and moderate eye by relaxing the oblique muscles suggests that the tension of the oblique muscles initiated a neurological change.

4.4.1   A RESTRICTION ON THE CILIARY MUSCLE OR LENS?

It makes a difference whether the restriction was imposed on the ciliary muscle or the crystalline lens. If the restriction was imposed on the ciliary muscle, it would suggest an indirect relationship between the oblique muscles and the ciliary muscle with the regulatory role assigned to the oblique muscles. If the restriction was imposed on the crystalline lens, it would suggest that there is a direct relationship between the lens and the rectus muscles with the regulatory role assigned to the rectus muscles.

4.4.2   A RESTRICTION ON THE CILIARY MUSCLE

If the myopic eye is within the myopic model, there is an indirect restriction placed on the ciliary muscle by the oblique muscles. A neurological regulation accounts for the immediate corrections of the lens' myopic shape. There is no direct link between the ortho C lens and the crystalline lens. The "contact lens draw" by itself does not shorten the elongation of the eyeball and the lens. It needs to be combined with a "focal point draw" (as explained in the chapter *How It Reverses Nearsightedness*).

After the brain recognizes that the eye is in distant mode, the proper neurological message is sent to the ciliary muscle and the rectus muscles through the common cranial nerve C3. It is the motor cortex that reverses the deviation of the crystalline lens and eyeball in the proper proportion. You do not need one contact lens with a specific flatness intended for the crystalline lens and another lens with a specific flatness for the eyeball.

4.4.3   A RESTRICTION ON THE LENS

Doonan (1984) suggested that there is another type of restriction. There is a mechanical link between the crystalline lens and eyeball. The zonule fibers are responsible for determining the shape of the lens. The change in the axial length of the eyeball can alter the lens' shape by relaxing the zonule fibers.

According to the mechanical model, the lens became myopic due to the rectus muscles instead of the ciliary muscle. Once the rectus muscles relax due to myopia, for example, the eyeball elongates. The elongation causes the zonule fibers to become slack because the vertical distance across the middle of the eye decreases. The slack of the fibers between the lens and the ciliary muscle in turn causes the lens to bulge independent of the ciliary muscle.

A difficulty with the mechanical model is that the lens remains thin during the developmental stage as the axial length of the eye became longer during myopia (Mutti et al., 2012). The elongation of the eye does not exhibit the expected mechanical effect on the lens during development. The adverse effect of near-point stress on the developmental eye is that the thinning process came to a halt. It was supposed to continue as the eye normally became larger. Thus the development of the lens is neurologically incomplete. (Refer to the chapters *Extraneous Variables* and *Treating Progressive Myopia* for more information.)

Under those conditions, the ciliary muscle still became thick (Bailey et al., 2008). It seems that the myopic model (how the eye became myopic due to near-point stress) is still in effect. According to the mechanical model, the ciliary muscle should not have thicken; and the lens and eyeball should have bulged at the same time instead of only the eyeball.

4.5   IMPOSING A NEUROLOGICAL RESTRICTION

When stress is not directly induced, the excessive tension of the oblique muscles neurologically imposes a ceiling on how much the ciliary muscle can relax to allow the lens to flatten to make out something clearly far away. The tension of the oblique muscles does not cause the ciliary muscle to seize up. The bulged shape of the lens in the mild and moderate myopic eye within the myopic model is not due to ciliary muscle spasm. There is a restriction in how much the lens can flatten for the distance without inducing spasticity.

The ciliary muscle can still flex and relax. The crystalline lens can still bulge some more for near focusing, and it can still flatten out to a certain extent from its bulged shape for distant focusing (up to the ceiling imposed). It implies that there is a neurological or indirect stimulation. If spasm has set in, it implies that there is a direct stimulation.

The excessive tension of the oblique muscles is also not spastic tension. If spasm had set in, then the oblique muscles cannot carry their primary function, but the oblique muscles can still carry out their normal function even if your myopia is in the progressive myopic range. If spasticity had set in, you would experience a limitation in the eye's movement.

4.6   DEVELOPING THE THEORY BEHIND THE TREATMENT

4.6.1   THE PROBLEM

You need to know the problem before you can treat it. The treatment for myopia relies on the hypothesis in relation to the problem: the motor cortex regards the myopic eye to be in near focus mode due to the excessive tightness of the oblique muscles. It maintains the myopic shape of the crystalline lens and eyeball even when the object of regard is known to be far away.

The hypothesis can be demonstrated by applying an ortho C lens to relieve the excess tension of the oblique muscles. An ortho C lens is designed slightly flatter than the cornea. The flatness is only a fraction of the flatness of an ortho K lens to allow a "contact lens draw" to "loosen" the oblique muscles. The "contact lens draw" also depends on a "focal point draw" before the oblique muscles can sufficiently relax. Once the lens relaxes the tension of those muscles by the proper amount, it also relaxes the tension of the ciliary muscle (to flatten out the lens) and increases the tension of the rectus muscles (to reduce the elongation of the eyeball). It presupposes that prior to the treatment, the excessive tension of the oblique muscles had maintained the myopic shape of the lens and eyeball.

4.6.2   THE CAUSE

The treatment for myopia also relies on the order of how the emmetropic eye became myopic. According to the theory behind near-point stress, the lens deviated first before the eye takes on an elongated shape. Thus the treatment needs to target the crystalline lens first and then the eyeball. The myopic lens must flatten first before the myopic eye can retract. It is based on how myopia set in and how the eyeball became elongated. In every drill proposed in the following chapters, relaxing the oblique muscles must attend to the crystalline lens first and then to the eyeball. You cannot ignore the lens and attempt to exclusively reverse the eyeball. Otherwise the treatment would not work.

The following phenomenon further reinforces the premise that the eyeball cannot retract unless the crystalline lens reverses first. If spasticity had set in, it would affect the ciliary muscle. Wearing glasses for all ocular ranges would induce it. It displaces the myopic eye outside the myopic model. If the resistance is partial, the patient needs to perform different resistance tests to find which drill can unlock the tension of the ciliary muscle before the eyeball retracts. If there is a total resistance, none of the proposed drills can relieve the tension of the ciliary muscle; as a result, the eyeball remains elongated.

KEYWORDS

- emmetropic eye
- myopic eye
- myopic shape
- cranial nerve
- extraocular muscles
- mechanical regulation
- neurological regulation

CHAPTER 5

THE MYOPIC MODEL

ABSTRACT

Ortho C is most effective when the patient's myopia is within the myopic model. An important characteristic that differentiates myopia within the myopic model from myopia outside the model is that the crystalline lens can still change its curvature (within the limits imposed by the tension of the oblique muscles). The tension induced by the oblique muscles places a limitation on how much the ciliary muscle can relax, but it does not compromise the muscle's flexibility. It is an indication that spastic tension was not induced. It allows a "focal point draw" to flatten the myopic crystalline lens before the elongated eyeball can retract—according to the theory behind the treatment for myopia.

The patient's nearsightedness is within the myopic model if it has the following features:

- It was due mainly to near-point stress.
- There are no other offsetting factors contributing to the eye's deterioration—such as wearing minus lenses for the near and midrange as well as for the distance.
- The onset of myopia is preferably in the postdevelopment stage.

The assumption is that patients with mild or moderate myopia are subjected to less extraneous variables. They are not necessarily immune from certain bad habits; rather, there is no need to engage in them—such as wearing their prescription glasses all the time. By not engaging in those habits, their eyes are in a more correctable state compared to someone else with higher ranges of myopia. So on the one hand, the conditions of the myopic model are undesirable because they are responsible for nearsightedness; but on the other hand, those conditions permit the ortho C lenses to work.

Thus what I am doing is not just matching ortho C to the problem but also the problem to ortho C. To determine the eye's resistance to ortho C, you would conduct a resistance test as outlined in the chapter *The Theory Behind the Resistance Tests*. Also refer to the chapter *The Procedure* for the context surrounding the tests.

5.1   FLEXIBILITY OF THE CILIARY MUSCLE

An important characteristic that differentiates myopia within the myopic model from myopia outside the model is that the crystalline lens can still change its curvature. The tension induced by the oblique muscles places a limitation on how much the ciliary muscle can relax, but it does not compromise the muscle's flexibility. The ciliary muscle can still alternatingly flex and relax. It can still tense up for close-up focusing and relax again to a certain extent (within the limits imposed by the tension of the oblique muscles) for distant focusing. It is an indication that spastic tension was not induced.

I depend on the flexibility of the ciliary muscle to kick start the reversal of the eyeball as well as the lens. As the lens starts to flatten, the elongated eyeball will eventually follow suit—as emphasized in the chapter *The Theory Behind the Resistance Tests*. It is the opposite of near-point stress. As the lens flattens as much as possible, it activates the eyeball to flatten to alleviate the extra work imposed on the ciliary muscle.

5.2   THE IMPACT OF A MINUS LENS

Another important feature of the myopic model is that the eye became myopic on its own accord. It took place naturally. The tension of the ciliary muscle was indirectly induced. If the tension of the ciliary muscle was directly induced, it would interfere with the flexibility of the lens. One of the ways stress is directly imparted to the ciliary muscle is by constantly wearing a minus lens for all ocular ranges. The overcorrection causes the ciliary muscle to tighten up to its maximum and the lens to bulge to its maximum. The tension of the oblique muscles increases so that the eyeball can elongate to alleviate the stress since the focal point is behind the retina.

In general, mild or moderate myopia is usually more receptive to ortho C compared to midrange or severe myopia. There is the tendency for mild and moderate individuals to refrain from relying on minus lenses for the near and midrange as well as for the distance. However, you may still come across some patients wearing their glasses all the time with the erroneous belief that it would curb their nearsightedness. You would not just be dealing with myopia. You also have to deal with progressive myopia, a loss of depth perception, or both. Those are separate problems by themselves.

5.3   DEVELOPMENT AND POSTDEVELOPMENT

When near-point stress takes place concurrently with another adverse condition, the extraneous variable is not necessarily a negative feature per se; rather it is an adverse feature in respect to hindering the desired outcome. The development of the eye, for example, is an important process; but when it occurs concurrently with near-point stress, the myopic eye becomes different.

The difficulty with the onset of myopia during development lies in the shape the crystalline lens assumes in response to near-point stress. The lens does not bulge as much (Mutti et al., 2012). There is less room for the lens to flatten out in response to ortho C. The eyeball tends to inherit more of the myopia to compensate for the lens' inability to bulge sufficiently at the near range. It is more difficult to stimulate the eyeball to shorten compared to the lens. In some cases, however, the Modified Preliminary Drill can be successful in correcting youths with high myopia during development. It is another area I am researching further for a future publication on dealing with difficult cases of myopia.

In the interim, your client would be more responsive to ortho C if mild or moderate myopia set in during postdevelopment. Once the eye ceases to elongate developmentally, the eyeball puts up a higher resistance to myopia and tends to elongate less compared to the lens. The crystalline lens bulges more during the onset of myopia to absorb most of the myopia. There is more room to flatten out in response to ortho C. It is easier to entice the lens to "shift" compared to the eyeball.

The age of the patient and when the onset of myopia took place are important considerations when screening clients to determine whether ortho C is suitable for them. It is comparable to assessing a client's suitability for laser surgery. (Refer to the chapter *Treating Progressive Myopia* for more information.)

5.4   IT DEPENDS ON THE PROBLEM

It is easier to treat hyperopia instead of myopia during development. With hyperopia the lens assumes most, if not all, of the deviated shape. I would just entice the lens to bulge instead of the lens and eyeball. The drill is simpler and is performed less often for maintenance. My youngest participant was 5 years of age with hyperopia of +2.50 in both eyes. I improved her vision to the extent where she only visits me once every 2 months and then gradually once every 4 months. The intention is not just to improve her visual acuity further but to maintain it by reestablishing the synchronization between the lens and eyeball.

KEYWORDS

- myopic model
- mild myopia
- hyperopia
- moderate myopia
- bad habits
- development
- postdevelopment

CHAPTER 6

EXTRANEOUS VARIABLES

ABSTRACT

I allowed for certain extraneous variables in a controlled environment. It permits you to conduct a Wearing Sequence Test and Resistance Test. A decrease in visual acuity may occur, but it is temporary. There are other extraneous variables which have a more lasting effect. The patient should learn about them to avoid a relapse.

6.1 THE PREFERRED RANGE

Initially I wanted to write about the treatment for hyperopia (and presbyopia). It is easier to treat hyperopia (even presbyopia) compared to myopia. The deviation is mainly attributed to the crystalline lens. Later I realized that such a book may not be appreciated unless I first reveal the difficulties in treating myopia. (The treatment for hyperopia is based on the treatment for myopia.)

It took me over 30 years to gather all the information for treating different types of nearsightedness. To make it manageable so that you can relate it to the theory behind the treatment, I decided to write about dealing with mild and moderate cases first. Those ranges of myopia are exposed to less extraneous variables compared to the higher ranges. The patient does not necessarily become immune to some of them; rather, there is no need to adopt some of those habits. For example, it is not necessary to rely on glasses all the time. The "effort to see" and mental strain in this range is less.

6.2 WHAT ABOUT THE INDEPENDENT VARIABLE?

The counterargument is that besides the dependent variable (the myopic eye), an extraneous variable can also affect the independent or manipulating variables (the proposed drills and the design of the lens). I have considered that possibility in *Verification*. In that section, I based the success of the treatment on the reliability of the method and the standard design of the lens—and on arguments why the outcome is due to neurology.

6.3   TESTS IN A CONTROLLED ENVIRONMENT

6.3.1   THE WEARING SEQUENCE TEST

I allowed for a possible negative outcome during a Sequence Test. The patient has to wear one lens at a time starting with the weaker eye. You may already have a hint which eye is the weaker eye from the prescription and the visual acuity test. The Wearing Sequence Test would confirm it. (Refer to the chapter *The Procedure* for more information.)

Do not be alarm if the patient's vision became blurred after the test. Suppose after wearing the right lens to perform a drill, the binocular visual acuity improved by one line on the Snellen chart; but after wearing the left lens to perform the same drill, it deteriorated. The blurriness is only temporary, and it is an indication that the sequence is incorrect. In some cases, the better eye is not necessarily the eye with the lower prescription.

You can reset the patient's visual acuity by wearing the right lens again. The test indicates that you should wear the left lens first and the right lens afterwards—not the other way around. You have to finish with the better eye—not the weaker eye. I can make your vision clear or blur at will depending on which sequence is correct. It is another indication that the procedure involves a neurological component.

In almost all cases, one eye is better than the other. Regardless if the prescription for each eye is the same, you still have to determine which eye is better—or just slightly better. If you have the same prescription for both eyes, you can still determine the weaker eye by performing a visual acuity test. Often I can guess which eye is more receptive. It is usually the eye with the lower prescription. If the patient inadvertently performed the wearing sequence incorrectly, there would not be the standard two-line improvement on the Snellen chart even if the eye was receptive to ortho C. The theory behind the wearing sequence is that the binocular vision takes on the visual acuity of the eye that performed the drill last. If the participant reversed the sequence, the binocular vision takes on the lower visual acuity of the weaker eye instead of the better eye.

6.3.2 RESISTANCE TESTS

There are also resistance tests which you would have the patient conduct in a controlled environment to determine the eye's resistances. A low resistance means the eye is receptive to ortho C. A partial resistance implies a less than expected response. It is possible for an eye to be within the myopic model and have a partial resistance. It falls under the category of secondary refractive errors—such as anisometropia and compound astigmatism. A secondary refractive error offers a resistance to the Standard Drill, but it can be treated by another type of drill designed for the specific problem. An eye can also put up a partial resistance when it falls slightly outside the myopic model. Most likely near-point stress was induced directly instead of indirectly. If the patient did something out of the ordinary such as wearing glasses for the near range as well as for the distance, the eye would incur a higher resistance to ortho C. The resistance tests would pick up both types of partial resistances. (The tests are described in the chapter *The Theory Behind the Resistance Tests*. Also refer to the chapter *The Procedure*.)

It is also possible for an eye to have a high resistance and show no response to the tests due to a more severe offsetting variable (or variables). I would inform participants with a high resistance that if they still decide to proceed, they would have to deal with certain habits first prior to the treatment. For example, if they wore glasses all the time, I would tell them to remove them whenever possible and to relax the ciliary muscle by performing certain relaxation drills. With mild and moderate myopia, it is possible for the ciliary muscle to become sufficiently relaxed in a couple of weeks. With severe myopia, it would take longer. In some cases, atrophy reinforces the spasm. (Refer to the chapter *Treating the Loss of Depth Perception* for more information.)

6.4 EXTRANEOUS VARIABLES OUTSIDE A CONTROLLED ENVIRONMENT

When the client leaves the controlled environment, I cannot observe the impact from other possible types of extraneous variables on the outcome from the treatment. The only way I can determine their presence is to rely on the visual acuity tests and on the patient's narrative during a follow-up. If the patient's visual acuity relapsed somewhat, most likely a negative factor was induced directly instead of indirectly; on top of that, it was probably induced unnaturally instead of naturally to produce ciliary muscle spasm. In some cases, however, the eye may inherit natural offsetting conditions on top of near-point stress, and that can hamper the retention.

6.5   INDIRECT INDUCTION

If the ciliary muscle was indirectly affected by near-point stress and if the prescription is in the mild or moderate range, the refractive error is likely within the myopic model. It can be verified by performing a Resistance Test. The ciliary muscle's flexibility is a leading indicator of the resistance of the eye. A high flexibility suggests that the tension of the oblique muscle was passed onto the ciliary muscle indirectly in terms of limiting how much the ciliary muscle is capable of relaxing. The effect of near-point stress was indirectly induced.

If it was directly induced, the contraction of the ciliary muscle would be seized; and the lens would be immobilized in a bulged shape. It is more difficult for ortho C to deal with directly induced stress than indirectly induced stress. The former also causes a loss of depth perception. (Refer to the chapter *Treating the Loss of Depth Perception* for more information.)

6.6   DIRECT INDUCTION

There is a strong correlation between near-point stress and your patient's initial myopic state (Dirani et al., 2008a). Near-point stress indirectly induces tension by placing a limitation on how much the ciliary muscle can relax. If the tension was directly imparted to the ciliary muscle, another negative variable was introduced in addition to near-point stress. The additional negative factor (or factors) can push it outside the myopic model by inducing spasticity instead of imposing a restriction.

6.6.1   WEARING A MINUS LENS INDISCRIMINATELY

A common extraneous variable is wearing a minus lens indiscriminately for all distances. As a result, the ciliary muscle can become seized in a bulged shape. The induction of stress on the ciliary muscle was transmitted directly. Even if the patient wore a weaker prescription, the focal point is still behind the retina when the object of regard is close-up or in the midrange. The light rays in that range are divergent. A minus lens causes the light rays to diverge more. The crystalline lens has to bulge more to bring it back onto the retina. The oblique muscles would attempt to alleviate the stress by tightening up to force the eye to elongate but then spasticity would tend to set in. The result would eventually be a loss of depth perception, horizontally and vertically. (Refer to the chapter *Treating the Loss of Depth Perception* for more information.)

6.6.2   NEGATIVE VARIABLES DUE TO THE METHOD

So far the extraneous variables mentioned are related to the dependent variable: the myopic eye. There are also extraneous variables that affect the independent variable or the variables that are manipulated: the drills and the ortho C lens. For example, the patient may have performed the drill incorrectly. You have to backtrack to ensure that the steps are adhered to exactly. If the first part of the Standard Drill was performed with the weaker eye first, for example, the outcome would be different. I have addressed such issues in Part 3 of the book on *Verification*.

6.7   UNNATURAL INDUCTION

6.7.1   BY A MINUS LENS

If the ciliary muscle was directly affected, often the stimulation was induced unnaturally. The ciliary muscle became seized independent of the influence of the oblique muscles. Again, an example of such a negative variable would be wearing a minus lens while the eye was engaged in near work. There would be a greater chance for spasm to set in. The directly induced stress from a minus lens is greater than indirect induced stress when bringing into focus the same object of regard. The focal point is farther behind the retina, and it affects the crystalline lens directly. The oblique muscles cannot immediately force the eyeball to elongate that much to alleviate the stress. Initially, the lens would have to bear the burden. It is easier for the lens to bulge than the eyeball.

6.7.2   BY APPLYING ANOTHER METHOD

The application of a different method may not work in conjunction with ortho C. If you apply plus lens therapy, for example, it can flatten the lens—but in a different way. Although it manages to stimulate the intra-ocular muscle to produce the correct outcome for distant focusing, it interferes with how the proper message relates to a distant object. Ortho C flattens the lens for distant focusing by attempting to reinstate the correct neuromuscular message to relax the ciliary muscle. Plus lens therapy attempts to flatten the lens by forcing the ciliary muscle to relax when regarding an image in the close range. Both eyes are directed inwards since the object of regard is close-up.

The depth perception of a myopic eye informs the visual cortex that the image of regard is near, but the ciliary muscle is forced to relax before the image can clear up due to the change in the rays of light by the plus lens. The rays became parallel as if the object is far away. It is contrary to how the ciliary muscle is supposed to behave when the object of regard is up close.

The other problem is that the client applies an excessive "effort to see." The effort is continuous. The eyeball cannot shorten to relieve the effort imposed on the ciliary muscle because the oblique muscles are still tight. All the correction is restricted to the crystalline lens. If the patient performed ortho C afterwards, the "contact lens draw" would not activate a "focal point draw." The neurological message created by the plus lens conflicts with the correct message.

6.8   NATURAL INDUCTION

The natural induction of stress is usually within the myopic model. It is natural in the sense that the patient did not wear a minus lens to make it more difficult to bring an object into focus in the near or midrange. There are instances, however, when the natural induction from near-point stress displaces the myopia outside the myopic model.

6.8.1   MYOPIA DURING DEVELOPMENT

If myopia occurred during development, it would interfere with ortho C. The onset of myopia brings the developmental process to a halt instead of causing the crystalline lens to bulge. According to research, the lens' neutral shape is thinner than the emmetropic eye. You cannot flatten it out more for the distance. The inflexibility of the lens at the close range contributes to progressive myopia once myopia sets in by failing to provide a braking mechanism to slow down the elongation of the eye. Thus most of the myopia may reside in the eyeball. (Refer to the chapter *Treating Progressive Myopia* for more information.)

6.8.2   *MYOPIA ACQUIRED BY GENETIC DISPOSITION*

There could be a genetic disposition relating to the onset of myopia during postdevelopment. According to Dirani et al.'s (2008) study of 612 twin pairs, myopia due to the quest for higher education is strongly influenced by genes. The participants were 18 years of age or older. The authors mentioned that the quest for higher education is strongly influenced by genes and is not strictly an environmental risk factor. The same genetic factors that influence an individual's education may also be involved in the development of that individual.

Although there is the propensity to become myopic, I think the influence of genetics resides in the background. It still has to be activated. I have seen cases where the encouragement of good habits can prevent the onset of myopia. The siblings had perfect eyesight while their parents are highly myopic. Throughout grade school and high school, they were constantly encouraged by their parents to look away at certain intervals when they were consistently performing near work. They were also constantly reminded to maintain a certain distance from the printed page.

They ended up at university taking challenging programs such as engineering and science and still maintain perfect vision when those habits became intact. I have checked their eyesight and found that at high school, their vision was better than normal. By the time they finished university, their vision is still good. It was not as good as when they were in high school, but it was still 20/20.

Myopia due to genetics is not necessarily more challenging to correct. I had cases where the mother with moderate myopia was easy to treat; and the moderate myopia of her daughters also had less resistance to ortho C. I also had cases where the mother with severe myopia was easy to "reduce," but her son's severe myopia was more difficult to treat, even though he was persistent in attempting to reduce it.

I had teens whose myopia were as high as their parents, and they were initially responsive to ortho C; but they later became less responsive due to their behavior and attitude. Their lack of seriousness in the treatment allowed negative variables to creep in. They seem to adapt their parents' behavior. If the mother is indifferent about her myopia, for example, then the sibling also tends to be indifferent—despite the mother's interest in the sibling's well-being.

6.9   OTHER TYPES OF EXTRANEOUS VARIABLES

The follow are some other extraneous variables that are more subtle and are difficult to categorize:

- The interference from mental strain.
- Continuously making an excessive "effort to see."
- Failing to "let go" when an image is blur or partially blur.

I will go over these adverse variables in the following chapters. All the extraneous variables mentioned are by no means complete. I am sure others will surface, but the key is that we can learn from them. I agree we do not have absolute knowledge as to what constitutes a successful treatment. I think that the more we uncover the conditions which can trigger a relapse and figure out how to deal with them, the more stable the outcome from ortho C.

6.10   WHEN A NEGATIVE VARIABLE CAN OCCUR

The patient needs to realize that negative factors can interfere at any time. It does not necessarily occur just during the onset of myopia. It can also occur after an improvement in visual acuity. You would find the same phenomenon in laser surgery. It is common for the patient's visual acuity to regress. A number of extraneous variables were not addressed. The oblique muscles are still very tight, the ciliary muscle is still tense, and the rectus muscles tension is incorrect. There is still the tendency for the lens or eyeball to deviate due to near-point stress.

6.11   ORTHO C AND LASER SURGERY

You may question the effectiveness of ortho C if it cannot stand up to certain extraneous variables, but even laser treatment is vulnerable to them. If your vision starts to regress after you had laser treatment and if you wore a minus lens all the time to address it, for example, the regression would become worse. The initial regression prior to resorting to any visual aid is common. The main culprit still exists after corrective surgery: the increase in tension of the oblique muscles. The eye is still vulnerable to the negative factors that can trigger the oblique muscles to tighten up more.

I am not criticizing laser surgery. I think it is an ingenious application of a laser to correct certain ranges of nearsightedness. Dr. Peyman, the inventor of LASIK, acknowledged the limitations of his invention and patented other means to improve it. I am sure he would have considered ortho C as a possible complementary process. I have numerous clients whose vision started to regress after they had laser surgery. Ortho C offered them another option. Instead of shaving more off the cornea during a touch-up, ortho C enhanced their visual acuity by attending to the source of the problem.

6.12   ADOPT GOOD HABITS

One way to counter extraneous variables that are due to bad habits is to practice good habits to offset them. The following are some habits the patient should adopt:

- Get into the habit of accepting a blur distant object. It is a subtle way of refraining from trying to force it into focus when it cannot come into focus or to maintain its clarity when it is difficult to do so. (Refer to the chapter *Letting Go* for more information and to the TV drill designed to speed up the saccadic movement in the *Addendum.*)
- Avoid wearing your prescription glasses for close-up work—even your weaker glasses. You only need them for driving and for temporarily making something out in the distance. A minus lens is not designed for reading. It causes the rays of light to diverge

more, and the crystalline lens will have to bulge more before an object can come into focus.

- Avoid wearing glasses when working in the intermediate range—such as wearing them to view the computer screen or the TV. Light rays from those ranges are still divergent. The minus lens diverges the rays even more. The crystalline lens will then have to bulge more before an object can come into focus.

- Frequently adjust the near or reading range until it is 14 or 16 in. away until it becomes a habit. (Refer to the Stretching Drill in the chapter *The Effort to See* and in the *Addendum.*)

- Frequently adjust the midrange or computer range until it is about 20 in. away until it becomes a habit. (Refer to the stretching drill in the chapter *The Effort to See* and in the *Addendum.*)

- Wear glasses instead of contact lenses. You cannot take the contact lenses off as easily as glasses when you finished viewing what you want to make out in the distance.

- Break the habit of overworking your eyes—such as reading for hours at a stretch without pause. Consider what happened after you wore the ortho C lenses for the first time. The improvement in visual acuity only took a few minutes. Although it is the opposite of what would happen if you were exposed to near-point stress, it still gives you an idea of how easy it is to alter your vision. Get into the habit of utilizing the 20/20 rule: every 20 min, look beyond 20 ft for 20 s.

- Place more emphasis on the "clarity" of an object as oppose to its "sharpness." You tend to equate that "sharpness" with what you see with your full prescription, but that prescription is likely overcorrected.

- Whenever possible, adjust or modify the conditions of your surroundings. For example, you can dim the lights to avoid glare, choose natural light over artificial light, or combine them both by moving closer to a window that allows an adequate source of natural light.

- If you cannot improve your surroundings, you can try to adapt to them when you are engaged in extensive close-up work. For example, you can look away momentarily when your eyes become too tired, or you can relax your eyes by closing them momentarily, perform the palming drill, etc.

- Break the habit of squinting when you cannot make something out in the distance. Instead, get into the new habit of "letting go" of it. You will consciously do it at first. Later it becomes a habit.

6.13   A LEARNING COMPONENT

Although the treatment only takes minutes instead of days or months, you have to remind the patient that there is also a learning component. The patient has to learn how to insert and remove the lenses. If the initial discomfort produces a lot of tears due to an overly sensitive cornea, it can interfere with the expected outcome. The patient may not experience a maximum improvement until a certain comfort level is gained. (The information on insertion and removal is given in the *Addendum*.) The patient needs to learn the proposed drill and perform the steps exactly. You have to emphasize adhering to protocol. The patient must recognize the extraneous variables that can induce a relapse, etc.

KEYWORDS

- **extraneous variable**
- **dependent variable**
- **independent variable**
- **controlled environment**
- **indirect induction**
- **direct induction**
- **unnatural induction**

CHAPTER 7

MENTAL STRAIN

ABSTRACT

Your memory is also myopic once you became nearsighted. The memory of your myopic state needs to be reconstructed along with your nearsightedness. The imprint of a blur object when your myopia was at its worse replaces your memory of its sharpness when your vision was normal. When you see something blur in the distance, you respond by reaching out for some sort of visual aid.

Mental strain is a hidden extraneous variable. It can prevent you from acknowledging an improvement in visual acuity by blocking the expectation to see better. It poses a barrier to any natural treatment which just relies on relaxation exercises.

The speed and degree of the initial improvement differentiates ortho C from other means of natural treatment by "shocking" your memory. It is possible for the instant clarity in vision to break the mental barrier that doubts the possibility of an actual improvement. The pronounced improvement can offset your myopic memory.

7.1 IT BLOCKS THE REALIZATION OF AN IMPROVEMENT IN VISION

My nearsightedness started when I was in grade four. The awareness of my deficiency in vision from an early age had induced what I called "mental strain." I attributed it to my memory of a blur image when my visual acuity was at its worse.

Before I discovered ortho C, I managed to reduce my nearsightedness by applying certain natural relaxation drills and by relying less on my glasses and contact lenses. I resorted to an undercorrected pair of glasses only for emergencies. I did not realize the implications of the improvement in my visual acuity—maybe because it was gradual. It took such a long time. Although my vision was much better compared to what it used to be, it was still not within the range where it convinced me that I reduced my nearsightedness considerably. At one time, my myopia was as high as −10.00 D (which was mainly due to edema from the nonoxygen permeable polymethyl methacrylate contact lenses). The mental block was a constant reminder that my nearsightedness was still the norm.

It prevented me from realizing how much my vision improved. Although I passed the vision test for my driver's license, I was not impressed. I should have been ecstatic, but I still see things slightly blur. So I thought the improvement was not that significant. I was not aware of the difference between how a blur object appears when I was −10.00 D compared to a blur object when I was 20/40. It seemed that mental strain blocked the realization of the extent of my improvement—even though it was mainly attributed to the crystalline lens.

7.2   YOUR MYOPIC MEMORY

Your memory, as well as your eye, is subjected to a refractive error once you become nearsighted. Suppose your myopia progressed to severe myopia. The memory of that myopic state has to be reconstructed along with your nearsightedness. The imprint of the blurriness of a distant object when your nearsightedness was at its worse replaces your memory of its sharpness when your vision was normal.

You are also reinforcing your myopic memory by remembering the sharpness of a distant object when you have your glasses on. So when you see something blur in the distance, you respond by reaching out for some sort of visual aid. You have accepted your nearsightedness as the norm, and you are not supposed to bring a distant object into focus without any visual aid.

When the normal eye sees something blur, it sends a neurosensory message to the motor cortex; and it responds by relaying a neuromotor message to the ciliary muscles to bring it into focus. The image will come into focus so fast that you were not conscious that the object was blur in the first place. If an image happens to remain blur, the normal eye would merely ignore it. It does not keep trying to bring it into focus.

7.3   YOUR MYOPIC MEMORY CAN OFFSET A CORRECTED EYE

Your myopic memory can create a resistance against acknowledging an improvement in vision. I once corrected a participant who had mild myopia by means of ortho C, but he subconsciously refused to acknowledge his corrected vision even though he could see down to line 9 on the Snellen chart. (Line 8 is the 20/20 line.) I reminded him that it is more difficult to gain a two-line improvement along the bottom half of the chart compared to the top half, but he continues to put on his full prescription glasses out of habit even when he did not need 20/20 vision to get by in his day-to-day activities. It was not due to a lack of knowledge of optometry. He was a health care professional. Perhaps his habit was reinforced by his myopic memory despite the immediate correction by ortho C. Thus he had to overcome a habit as well as mental strain.

The memory of the sharpness of a distant image created by a corrective lens or a corrective procedure can also impose a cognitive barrier. I had reduced the moderate myopia of another participant who had a partial resistance. He had attempted ortho K, and I told him to discontinue wearing the lenses for a month to allow the cornea to resume its former shape and to ease the spasticity of the ciliary muscle. Although he acknowledged an improvement in visual acuity from −1.75 to −0.75 after he performed the Standard Drill a few times, he preferred to go back to ortho K. The argument was that he was able to see 20/20 without glasses after ortho K. It overrode the logic why a weaker prescription was a better option to maintain his improvement in vision.

7.4   REVIVING THE REALIZATION OF THE EXTENT OF IMPROVEMENT

When the patient's memory is not severely myopic, the speed and degree of the initial improvement differentiates ortho C from other means of natural treatment for mild and moderate myopia. It "shocks" your memory in the sense that your memory of the instant clarity in vision is more pronounced than your myopic memory.

The sudden clarity in focus offsets a large portion of your mental strain. How much it offsets your myopic memory depends on how much your vision improved after the initial application. If there is a gain of two or three lines on the Snellen chart, there is a significant realization of an improvement in visual acuity. If there is just a one-line improvement, then there is only a partial realization of an improvement in visual acuity.

Weeks before the treatment, I would tell the participants who rely on their glasses a lot to depend on them less. By wearing them all the time, it places a higher restriction on how much the ciliary muscle can relax. Ortho C is not designed to deal with a loss of depth perception. It has to be dealt with separately. (Refer to the chapter *Treating the Loss of Depth Perception* for more information.) Even with severe myopia, just by removing the glasses and performing the relaxation, swinging, and stretching drills would make a difference in how much the eye can respond to ortho C. (Refer to the *Addendum* on how to perform those drills.)

7.5   REVIVING THE EXPECTATION TO SEE BETTER

The realization that there is an improvement leads to the expectation to see better. By performing the drill regularly, it preserves the improvement in visual acuity. Each time the patient performs the drill, he is actually "shocking" the visual system neurologically to see clearer. It reconstructs his myopic memory.

7.6   BELIEFS AND ATTITUDES

Encourage your patients to realize that they do not need 20/20 vision to get by in life. The severity of their mental strain is in direct proportion to the beliefs and attitudes about how they are supposed to accept the world around them. They are conditioned by their glasses or contact lenses to believe that they need perfect vision all the time, but they don't. It is the key reason why it is difficult to break bad habits such as wearing a minus lens to read when they do not have to.

There is the fear of "letting go" of such misconceptions. You have to explain to these patients that a minus lens is not intended for the near or intermediate range. Going about their day to day activities without glasses is also part of the treatment. The eyeball still needs to synchronize with the lens and one eye needs to synchronize with the other. (Refer to the chapters *Letting Go* and *Treating Progressive Myopia* for more information.)

KEYWORDS

- **mental strain**
- **myopic memory**
- **reinforcement**
- **resistance**

CHAPTER 8

THE EFFORT TO SEE

ABSTRACT

Most of the "effort to see" is due to bad habits. It includes habit such as constantly reading at an incorrect range, sitting too close to the computer, forcing a blur image to come into focus, and wearing a minus for all ocular ranges. Ortho C does not address the adoption of a bad habit, and it needs to be dealt with separately. One way to break an old habit is to replace it with a new habit.

8.1   AN EXCESSIVE EFFORT AT THE NEAR AND MIDRANGE

8.1.1   PRIOR TO THE TREATMENT

An "effort to see" is not just in reference to squinting to make something out far away. Even looking at a near object for an extended period can trigger an excessive "effort to see." It actually takes more effort for the emmetropic or normal eye to see something close than far away. The same can be said about the nearsighted eye even though its elongated shape can alleviate some of the effort.

The crystalline lens of a normal eye assumes a bulged or round shape to bring near objects into focus, and it flattens out to bring distant objects into focus. When focusing on an object close-up, the ciliary muscle becomes tense to expand the muscle—similar to how your biceps expand when you flex them. The reduction in the space between the ciliary muscle ring and the lens allows the zonule fibers, which connect the crystalline lens and the ciliary muscle ring around the lens, to become slack.

The lens will then bulge. It naturally strives to assume a round shape when the zonule fibers are not pulling on it. The closer the image, the tighter the ciliary muscle becomes to allow the fibers to become looser—and that in turn forces the lens to bulge more.

When you shift your focus to something far away, the ciliary muscle becomes relaxed. It constricts when it is in a relaxed state. The increase in space between the ciliary muscle ring and the lens allows the retraction to pull on the zonule fibers. The lens will then flatten out to bring a distant image into focus. Distant viewing takes place without any effort involved.

The initial deterioration in vision is usually due to an excessive effort to bring close-up objects into focus and to maintain it for an extended period. Most of us have perfect eyesight until we reach grade school. When we spent most of our time doing a lot of near work without taking a break, we become subjected to a specific type of "effort to see" that is sometimes referred to as "near-point stress."

Your reading range is normally considered to be 16 in. or 40 cm. When your daily routine involves work closer than 16 in., the crystalline lens would become more bulged. If an individual, especially during development, maintains such a curvature for an extended period without looking away now and then to relax the ciliary muscle, the lens may not snap back to its flat shape for distant focusing even if you look into the distance.

The increase in tension of the oblique muscles implies that the eye is in near focus mode (Yee, 2011). The brain treats a blur image in the distance as something that is blur close-up. If you made an excessive "effort to see" something in the distance, the oblique muscles would become tight with the intention to elongate the eyeball—as if though the eye was subjected to near-point stress. The excess tension was picked up by another part of the brain, and it short circuits the information received by your depth perception—that the object of regard is in the distance. The neuromotor message sent along the visual pathway directs the oblique muscles to become tighter instead of relaxed.

8.1.2   AFTER THE TREATMENT

The patient should be aware of any bad habits related to an increase in "effort to see." The myopic eye is still susceptible to them after it responds favorably to ortho C. To deal with the problem, the patient needs to learn to "let go" of a distant object once it comes into focus. Holding onto it out of habit tends to slow down the saccadic movement. (Refer to the chapter *Letting Go* for more information.)

8.1.3   ADJUST THE READING DISTANCE

After ortho C corrects the myopia, the patient may still look very close when bringing a near object into focus and thereby become subjected to near-point stress. He needs to alter the habit by consciously adjust the distance of regard until it falls 14 or 16 in. away. He may not maintain that range immediately but try to hold the "stretch" for just half a minute or so. Do not hold the focus too long in case it triggers an excessive "effort to see."

Just perform the "stretching" drill two or three times a day, and space it out accordingly. After the drill, allow the vision to settle back to its natural range which is a bit closer. The tendency to look closer is not necessarily to make the words clearer, but rather it is done out of habit. Later the natural range increases. The drill is more effective when it is done in conjunction with ortho C. (Refer to the *Stretching Drills* in the *Addendum* for more information.)

8.1.4   ADJUST THE MIDRANGE

The same idea applies to working in front of a computer screen. At first, sit at a comfortable distance in front of it. Then they would stretch their vision a bit by sitting farther away from it for about 5 min or so. Then they would go back to their normal range. Later, the normal range is adjusted.

The ideal distance is said to be 20 in. away, so try to maintain a distance between 16 and 20 in. away. How long it takes to make that adjustment depends on when they can break the habit of inching closer nd closer to the screen instead of maintaining a certain distance. (Refer to the *Stretching Drills* in the *Addendum* for more information.)

8.2   AN EXCESSIVE EFFORT DUE TO SQUINTING

During early onset, the nearsighted eye unlike the normal eye tends to make more effort to bring something far away into focus. It is in near focus mode for the distance as well as close-up. The amount of effort generated is more than what is normally required for distant focusing. There is the tendency to force an object into focus when it is a bit blur by narrowing the eyelids to alter the curvature of the cornea. Over time, squinting can induce corneal astigmatism (Yee, 2013a).

You may need to inform your clients if you notice any of them squeezing the upper and lower lids close together. Some of them may not realize that they are doing it. They may have to ask their friends or other members of their family to remind them not to squint whenever they notice it. They have to be aware of what the act of squinting feels like.

A reduction in squinting was reported by parents after I treated their siblings for severe myopia. A distant object is still partially blur during the initial stage, but they gradually refrained from squinting—even before they consciously try to break the habit. Perhaps the induction of "shock" was an important factor.

There may still be a certain degree of unconscious squinting which is manifested by a partial squint. The patient may not be aware of it; but onlookers from a certain angle will notice it. It is a good practice to open the eyes wide for about 10 s while repeating the reminder not to squint— even though there is no sign of squinting. Repeat the exercise now and then throughout the day. The "effort to see" is easier to control when the correct neuromuscular message is reinstated. To deal with any residual tendency to squint, similar to near-point stress, a certain amount of repetition is required to break the habit by replacing it with an alternative habit. When time permits, the palming drill afterwards. (Refer to the *Addendum* for information on palming.)

"Letting go" by watching TV is another effective technique. If the patient squints while watching a movie, it is done out of habit. Normally, the eye assumes a relaxed shape once the patient becomes immersed in the storyline. There is no urgency to make out different images sharply. The worse types of movies to watch are those with captions. Reading the captions forces the saccadic movement to slow down. It is accompanied by an increase in "effort to see" when the eye resists the natural tendency to take part in the movement on the screen.

After I improved the visual acuity of high myopic patients, they would find a distance in front of the TV where the "effort to see" is not so high that it triggers squinting. The TV is an effective tool to train them to "let go" and accept a blur object by increasing the saccadic movement according to how fast each frame changes.

When the eye moves from object to object, it breaks the urge to squint. It would consciously shift at first by looking at the different characters, their expression, the landscape, etc. Later, it would "let go" and explore once it adopts the new habit. (Refer to the section *Letting Go by Watching TV* in the *Addendum* for more information.)

8.3   AN EXCESSIVE EFFORT DUE TO MAINTAINING THE FOCUS OF A DISTANT IMAGE

There is also the tendency for the nearsighted eye to maintain the focus of a distant image longer than necessary. Forcing a blur image into focus by nudging the eye once or twice can take less effort than squinting, but holding that focus may take just as much effort as squinting. The patient may have experienced such a habit by trying to read something just outside the range where he can comfortably bring it into focus. He may find that he needs to expend 100% effort before he can read something on the blackboard or something projected onto a screen in a dim room. It means forcing the lens to adopt a maximum flat shape, but it bulges instead since the effort would become excessive. You cannot force the crystalline lens to flatten out. To prevent asthenopia (or eye strain), you need to expend 50% effort instead. (For more information on asthenopia, refer to the chapters *Letting Go* and *Treating Progressive Myopia*.)

A myopee can simulate the negative impact maintaining the "effort to see" can have on the myopic eye by regarding a letter on the Snellen chart that is slightly blur such as the "C" on the fifth line of the Snellen chart. To make it clearer, alternatingly look at the top part (to make the bottom blur) and then the bottom part (to make the top blur). By swinging the "C" steadily, the "C" as a whole becomes clear. Attempting to hold the clarity for 5 or 10 min in this manner, astigmatism can set in. When I did the experiment, the next day my colleague confirmed that the intense "effort to see" induced lenticular astigmatism (Yee, 2013b).

There are different variations of this technique to enhance your vision. They are not relaxation drills. They can be a form of squinting that affects the lens instead of the cornea. They are more like modification drills, but the problem is that you cannot force your vision to clear up. The effort would not relax the ciliary or oblique muscles.

8.4   AN EXCESSIVE EFFORT DUE TO FORCING A BLUR DISTANT IMAGE TO COME INTO FOCUS

If a patient has a partial resistance and there is still some residual myopia after ortho C, it is okay to wear a weaker pair of glasses for the distance. He may have attained the habit of not wearing any minus lenses for all ranges of ocular work. That is commendable. He should now extend the concept.

It is okay to wear a weaker prescription if he needs it to see something far away. The effort to bring a blur image into focus with the naked eye may result in an excessive effort to see. The glasses offset the effort it takes to bring a distant object into focus. By not wearing them for the blackboard or overhead, for example, it can compromise the improvement in vision due to another form of asthenopia: the strain from attempting to bring a blur object into focus when it is too blur. He would expend more than 100% effort. To prevent asthenopia, the amount of effort required should be 50% instead.

8.5   AN EXCESSIVE EFFORT DUE TO A MINUS LENS

Prescription glasses were intended to alleviate any excessive effort when attempting to make something out far away; but once you wear them all the time, another type of "effort" occurs. Similar to the act of squinting, you may not even be aware of it. A minus lens does not vary its focal length like the focal length of the crystalline lens when it considers objects at different distances. The crystalline lens of a myopic eye does not have any difficult bringing about near focusing, but distant focusing poses a problem because the focal length is too short. The fixed longer focal length of a minus lens would clear up a blur object in the distance; but it would be at the expense of affecting your near focusing since the focal length would be too long.

The eye chart is pegged at 20 ft during an eye test because light reaches the eye as parallel rays at that distance. Anything closer, the light rays diverges and the lens of your eye will have to bulge to shorten the focal length. A bulged or rounder crystalline lens converges the light rays so that the focal point will fall on the retina instead of behind it.

With a minus lens on, its concave shape diverges the light rays even more in the near and midrange. The crystalline lens can only bulge so much to converge the rays. The eyeball would come into play to alleviate the tension of the ciliary muscle when fatigue sets in during prolonged work. A certain amount of spasm already exists due to your nearsightedness. By inducing additional tension to bring a near image into focus, it further constricts the oblique muscles. The eye becomes longer from front to back to account for the minus lens' longer focal point. It is the only way it can bring an image in the close range into focus if the crystalline lens reached its maximum bulged shape.

You may argue that although you wear glasses all the time, you do not read that much; but most of your time is still spent in the midrange or closer throughout the day. If you work in an office, for example, you are probably confined to an area less than 20 ft all around. The only time you would look far away to allow the lens to flatten sufficiently is probably when you drive to work. You are focusing throughout the rest of the day on images close to you, like reading reports, "crunching" numbers, or working in front of a computer screen. The lens would bulge to bring them into focus in these ranges.

8.6   WEARING YOUR GLASSES ONLY FOR THE DISTANCE

It is okay to wear a weaker pair of minus lenses for the distance. The light rays are parallel, and that permits the focal point to be projected on the retina—not behind it as in overcorrected cases. That is why it is okay to drive for hours with a weaker pair of glasses. You are mainly focusing in the distance. Even though the prescription is undercorrected, the focal point is on the retina because under normal conditions, you are allowing a "focal point draw" to take place once it is reinstated neurologically. Also, the aperture of the eye is smaller—assuming that the weaker prescription was worn during the daytime when there is adequate natural light. The aperture opens less during the day than at night, and that allows a sharper image.

Ortho C activates a "focal point draw." Otherwise all you would need to do is wear a weaker pair of glasses with its focal point projected near the retina. There were researches attempting to induce a "draw" by such a process, but the difficulty lies in the first myopic relationship and the second myopic relationship. They were still intact. The correct neurological message was not reinstated to bring about the correct responses from the crystalline lens or the eyeball due to the tension of the oblique muscles. (Refer to the chapter *Neurological Implications* for more information on the first myopic relationship and the second myopic relationship.)

8.7   HOW LONG WOULD IT TAKE TO BREAK A BAD HABIT?

One way to break an old habit is to replace it with a new habit. You do not have to prolong the new repetition indefinitely. A new habit can be created by repeating it enough times (about 66 times). Missing a day or two would not change the habit; and extra repetitions beyond a certain point would not have an impact on automaticity (Lally et al., 2010). You would perform the repetitions consciously at first. Later, it becomes an unconscious activity.

KEYWORDS

- effort to see
- reading range
- computer range
- saccadic movement
- squinting

CHAPTER 9

LETTING GO

ABSTRACT

"Letting go" is the act of disengaging yourself from a specific object of regard in the distance and "moving on" to consider other objects in your visual field. Even after applying ortho C, it is a good idea to adopt the habit of "letting go" of everyday objects in the distance instead of constantly trying to make them out—especially if there is still some residual myopia. The myopee has to learn that not every blur object needs to be brought into focus. It takes too much effort to apply 100% of the lens' flexibility to bring a distant object into focus and then hold that focus. If it becomes a habit, it can offset some of the gains from ortho C. It can lead to asthenopia.

9.1 WHEN TO LET GO

There are two instances when you have to "let go" of an object:
- If it is too blur to bring into focus, and you keep pondering it to bring it into focus.
- If it comes into focus by applying 100% of the flexibility of the crystalline lens, and you want to hold that focus for an extended period.

9.2 WHY LET GO?

An excessive "effort to see" can trigger asthenopia. Donders suggested that the phenomenon is prevalent in cases of farsightedness (Grosvenor, 2007). It contributes to headaches since most of our day-to-day work is in the near and midrange. It is also a factor to consider after experiencing an improvement by ortho C. The excess effort stems from applying 100%

of the lens' flexibility to bring a distant object into focus. If it becomes a habit, it can offset some of the gains from ortho C. I would often remind my participants to get into the habit of "letting go" of an object within a certain period of time.

The advantage in performing the Preliminary Drill first before the Standard Drill is that you would learn how to get into the habit of "letting go" as well as learning to adapt to the lens. The excessive "effort to see" to bring a distant object into focus, by utilizing the total flexibility of the lens, can cause your improved visual acuity to fluctuate. The crystalline lens compensates for its own myopic shape and the myopic shape of the eyeball. The extra "load" is on top of any additional task involved such as calculating, taking notes, etc. The only way to minimize the fluctuation is to "let go."

The Preliminary Drill was mainly designed to treat anisometropia. You eventually have to perform the Standard Drill to reduce the eyeball's elongation, and that can reduce the "effort to see." The ability to control your "effort to see" when you are practicing with the Preliminary Drill will ensure that the effort is not excessive by the time you perform the Standard Drill.

Although your visual acuity would improve more by performing the Standard Drill first, you may still tend to engage in the habit of utilizing 100% of the crystalline lens to bring a distant object into focus. It is comparable to someone who is hyperopic and is in the habit of utilizing 100% of the crystalline lens' flexibility when performing close-up work. The rule is that you can only apply about 50% of the flexibility of the lens to avoid asthenopia. It is permissible to use most of the flexibility of the lens momentarily—but not to maintain this focus for an extended period.

9.3   LET GO OF AN OBJECT THAT IS TOO BLUR

Once you removed your glasses and try to get around as much as possible without them prior to ortho C, your work is cut out for you. There is the tendency for a moderate myopee to make an excessive "effort to see" to bring a blur object far away into focus.

You mainly want to get into the habit of "letting go" of an image that is too blur to bring into focus. Not every image causes your lens or eyeball to "shift." Only those objects whose focal points are projected close enough to the retina can activate a "focal point draw." An object that falls within that threshold is not so blur that it produce an excessive "effort to see"; instead, it is just blur enough to stimulate the lens to flatten to bring it into focus. But the myopic eye cannot immediately distinguish which images are too blur and which ones qualify for a "focal point draw." So you have to "let go" of every blur image instead of being selective.

9.4   CONSCIOUS OF A BLUR OBJECT

After the myopic eye fails to bring a blur object into focus, there is the tendency to make a conscious effort to bring it into focus. It slows down the saccadic movement which is an unconscious activity. When the saccadic movement is still intact, you would tend to "let go" of a blur object without you becoming aware of it. It scans from object to object at such a rate that the particular visual field as a whole is clear.

9.5   AVOID HOLDING A FOCAL POINT DRAW TOO LONG

If your severe myopia is within the myopic model, you may also have the habit of maintaining a "focal point draw" longer than necessary. The longer you try to hold an object in focus, the more you are extending the excessive "effort to see." Initially, the focal point of such an image did not fall onto the retina but in front of it, and the lens has to "shift" to bring it into focus. The crystalline lens may have to expend 100% of its flexibility to hold it in focus for an extended period. So what you are actually maintaining is its full flexibility. The wider the gap between the focal point and the retina, the more effort it takes, and the easier it is for fatigue to set in.

I am not saying that you should immediately "let go" or "move on" whenever a "focal point draw" brings an object into focus. Sometimes you have to make an assessment of a specific object. It takes more work, however, to constantly maintain as well as bringing into focus every object that comes into your visual field. It defeats the purpose of the saccadic movement.

It is interesting to note that you can maintain the focus of a distant image for an extended period if your "effort to see" and mental strain are at an acceptable level. It is no different than the effort utilized to sustain the focus of letters on a page held at a comfortable distance away. There is no excessive effort involved. Looking at distant objects in general is comparable to reading extensively without experiencing fatigue. The scanning rate is so quick that it considers the letters in segments. Each segment comes into focus so quick that it seems to come into focus at once.

9.6   AVOID INCREASING ITS SHARPNESS

9.6.1   INDIVIDUAL OBJECT

When you hold onto the focus of a distant image longer than necessary, the myopic eye also tends to make an excessive effort to "sharpen" it some more, but you cannot increase the "sharpness" of an object that is already in focus. Due to the eye's sluggish saccadic movement, the scanning rate is not fast enough to activate a "focal point draw" of every object in your field of vision. Their blurriness gives the impression that the individual object is still blur. If the saccadic movement was intact, it would give the impression that a group of objects come into focus all at once. A particular object selected from the group, however, would be more clear than the other objects.

9.6.2   GROUP OF OBJECTS

An object within a certain distance would come into focus by a "focal point draw," but groups of objects are still out of focus due to a sluggish saccadic movement. By forcing an increase in their "sharpness," it is another way of generating an excessive "effort to see." You may think that an object is not "sharp" because you are comparing an image which comes into focus by means of a focal point "draw" to groups of objects that failed to come into focus.

When your saccadic movement is functioning properly, central focusing takes place by zooming in on the images that you are scanning. Central focusing brings out the "sharpness" of a particular object while maintaining the "clarity" of the objects around it. It can also bring out the "sharpness" of a particular aspect of an object while maintaining the "clarity" of that object as a whole. When your saccadic movement is compromised, it is difficult to distinguish a particular object in your visual field or a particular aspect of an object.

When you look at a distant image with your glasses on, there is no "focal point draw" involved. The minus lens does all the work your eye muscles should be doing. The minus lens also replaced the eye's saccadic movement. It brings out the "sharpness" of every image before you instead of a particular image that you are focusing on. The minus lens also replaced how your central fixation normally works. It creates the illusion that every image is "sharp." It is an unnatural way to bring an object into focus. It does not differentiate between the "sharpness" of an object from the "clarity" of the other objects around it.

9.7   SPEED UP THE SACCADIC MOVEMENT

If you have severe myopia, your saccadic movement is sluggish. It contributes to the urge to bring every object in your visual field into focus—even when some are too blur. It adds to the excessive "effort to see" initiated by a specific object. If the "effort to see" increases, the saccadic movement would slow down even more. You would tend to become even more conscious of a blur image.

To break the habit, you have to consciously continue to "let go" of most blur images after you become conscious of them until it becomes an unconscious activity. You do that by accepting a blur object and by practicing certain relaxation drills such as palming and swinging. You also have to increase the rate you scan from object to object. The TV is actually a tool that can speed up the saccadic movement. You have to keeping up with the rate the picture changes on the screen. When the myopic eye's saccadic movement is brought up to speed, you will automatically relax and either allow a "focal point draw" to take place or ignore the object that is in question. (Refer to the *Addendum* for more information on the drill.)

9.8   ACCEPTANCE

"Letting go" of an object that is too blur implies acceptance. When you respond to a blur image by mentally accepting it, it is a subtle way of "letting go" after you became conscious of it. It takes less effort for the myopic eye to accept a blur image than to try to bring it into focus—after you became conscious of its blurriness.

When an object is not important enough to bring into focus, you have to consciously get into the habit of accepting it regardless if it is blur. If you accept it and do not have time to look away, you are still "letting go" of the urge to bring it into focus. It trains you to "let go" of images subconsciously—even if the saccadic movement is not up to par. Later it would be easier to "let go" of a blur image subconsciously once your saccadic movement improves.

When you learn to "let go" of a blur object, you are actually "letting go" of all ranges of blurriness—those that are indistinct as well as those that are not too blur and are qualified for a focal point "draw." By accepting an object as it is, it makes a "focal point draw" easier. You would also disregard the impulse to try to make it "sharper."

KEYWORDS

- asthenopia
- 100% flexibility
- 50% flexibility
- the Preliminary Drill
- the Standard Drill

CHAPTER 10

NEUROLOGICAL IMPLICATIONS

ABSTRACT

The most intriguing outcome after wearing an ortho C lens is the speed and degree of the initial improvement. When I began my research, I thought the treatment would be purely physiological. I came across the neurological implications by accident. My friend wanted to try ortho C and found that the lens which I inserted for him was irritating. I took it out with the intention of repositioning it on the cornea. He noticed that he could see clearer after I took it off. He only did the drill with the lens on for less than a minute.

At first, I thought it was still a physiological phenomenon, and it was due to the receptiveness of the eye. I had him wear the lenses longer and did the drills more frequently; but once he did that, his visual acuity was not as sharp as it was initially. He regained the sharpness after he reduced the wearing time while performing the drills. I realized that if the lens was worn too long, it would induce ortho K once the solution drains and the lens presses against the cornea instead of "drawing" on it. The deterioration in vision suggests that ortho C and ortho K do not mix.

Since it is possible to improve the visual acuity of the mild and moderate myopic eye in just a few minutes, it is an indication that neurology plays an important part in the reversal process. It is also an indication that neurology was involved in the problem. The excessive tension of the oblique muscles was responsible for the tension of the ciliary muscle and the slack of the rectus muscles.

10.1 NEUROLOGICAL RELATIONSHIP BETWEEN THE DIFFERENT MUSCLES OF THE EYE

There are neurological relationships between the different muscles of an eye that became nearsighted. If it is within the myopic model, the relationships can be verified by ortho C. When an ortho C lens reverses the crystalline lens' bulged shape by relaxing the oblique muscles, it exemplifies the first myopic relationship. When it also reverses the eyeball's elongated shape by relaxing the oblique muscles, it exemplifies the second myopic relationship. When it synchronizes the crystalline lens to the change in the shape of the eyeball, it demonstrates the third myopic relationship. And when it synchronizes the right and left eye, it demonstrates the fourth myopic relationship.

Neurology also plays a vital role in how the normal eye functions. There is a developmental relationship between the crystalline lens and the eyeball during childhood development and adult postdevelopment in the normal or emmetropic eye. Developmental factors determine the shape of the crystalline lens in relation to the eyeball, and postdevelopmental factors determine the shape of the eyeball in relation to the lens.

When the emmetropic eye brings day-to-day objects into focus, it activates a different neurological message. The eyeball does not change its shape to bring about near and distant focusing. The crystalline lens carries out that task. With sudden changes in focus from near to far and vice versa, only the ciliary muscle is flexible enough to facilitate the immediate changes. When immediate focusing is required, the lens acts independently. It is evident in mild myopia when the crystalline lens assumes a bulged shape first before the sclera starts to elongate to alleviate the stress incurred by the ciliary muscle.

On my website, however, I asked the following question: if the existing model for accommodation only involves the crystalline lens, then how did the eye become elongated? You need another model to explain it. The following are proposed theories of the myopic model.

10.2   THE DIFFERENT MYOPIC RELATIONSHIPS

10.2.1   NEUROLOGICAL RELATIONSHIP BETWEEN THE OBLIQUE MUSCLES AND CILIARY MUSCLE OF A MYOPIC EYE

The first theory is on the relationship between the oblique muscles and ciliary muscle of the myopic eye and its impact on the crystalline lens. The first myopic relationship can be expressed as follows: the excessive tension of the oblique muscles causes the ciliary muscle to become tense to entice the crystalline lens to bulge.

The first part of the Preliminary Drill presuppose that such a condition exists. The drill would not work if it did not exist. If the "contact lens draw" relaxes the oblique muscles, the ciliary muscle should also relax to allow the crystalline lens to flatten for distant focusing.

The tension of the oblique muscles and ciliary muscle is comparable to the neurological relationship between, for example, the right lateral rectus muscle and left medial rectus muscle when both eyes turn to the right. Both those muscles simultaneously become tense before the eyes can turn together. This is referred to as Hering's Law (Chornell et al., 2010). Perhaps the tension of the oblique muscles initiates a dual relationship between the oblique muscles and ciliary muscle that resembles a variation of Hering's Law.

The first myopic relationship comes into play when the ciliary muscle becomes very tight to maintain the maximum bulged shape of the crystalline lens for an extended period—when the object of regard is very close. The oblique muscles would be on standby to alter the shape of the sclera if necessary to alleviate the tension of the ciliary muscle during prolonged near focusing. If the increase in tension of the oblique muscles is not maintained, the ciliary muscle can still relax to flatten the lens for distant focusing.

However, once the excessive tension of the oblique muscles sets in, the brain would regard the eye to be stuck in near-focus mode. It gives precedence to the neurosensory message of the extra tension of the oblique muscles instead of a blur image. The tension of the ciliary muscle then becomes an extension of the tension of the oblique muscles. The excessive tension of the oblique muscles is the determining factor for the shape of the lens during distant focusing instead of the ciliary muscle.

It was the tension of the ciliary muscle due to near-point stress that initially influenced the oblique muscles to tighten up and the rectus muscles to relax to allow for a possible elongation of the sclera. When the ciliary muscle initiated this function, it is a sign that a change in regulatory role is pending. The tension of the oblique muscles induces a different type of tension onto the ciliary muscle. The fixed tension of the oblique muscles imposes a limit as to how much the ciliary muscle can flatten the crystalline lens for distant focusing (Yee, 2014).

The restriction placed on the lens is not due to the spasm of the ciliary muscle. The tension of the oblique muscles does not exactly cause the ciliary muscle to spasm. If spasticity was induced, the contraction of that muscle would be seized; but the ciliary muscle can still tense up some more for close-up focusing and relax again to a certain extent for distant focusing.

Instead of inducing spasticity, the tension of the oblique muscles neurologically imposes a ceiling on how much the ciliary muscle can relax (and thus how much the lens can flatten out) when trying to make something out in the distance. The restriction does not compromise the ciliary muscle's ability to tighten up further to allow the crystalline lens to bulge some more for near focusing. During early onset, the lens can also flatten to a certain degree due to its free play to bring a distant object into focus.

10.2.2 NEUROLOGICAL RELATIONSHIP BETWEEN THE OBLIQUE MUSCLES AND RECTUS MUSCLES OF A MYOPIC EYE

The second theory is on the relationship between the oblique muscles and the rectus muscles of the myopic eye and its impact on the sclera. The second myopic relationship can be stated as follows: the excessive tension of the oblique muscle causes the rectus muscles to relax to allow the eyeball to elongate.

The application of the first part of the Standard Drill to treat moderate myopia presupposes that the relationship exists. The drill would not work if it did not exist. If the "contact lens draw" relaxes the oblique muscles, the rectus muscles should tighten up to allow the eyeball to retract for distant focusing.

The eyeball as well as the crystalline lens is affected as the eye progresses to the higher ranges of myopia. The erroneous neuromotor message is relayed to the rectus muscles as well as the ciliary muscle. The rectus muscles come into play by offering enough slack to allow the eye to elongate. The eyeball becomes myopic when the tension of the rectus muscles does not oppose the oblique muscles' increased tension around the middle of the eyeball (Yee, 2011).

The tension of the oblique muscles and the relaxation of the rectus muscles are comparable to the neurological relationship between, for example, the right medial rectus muscle and the right lateral rectus muscle, for example, when the right eye turns to one side: one muscle must relax to allow the tension of the other muscle to turn the eye in that direction. This is referred to as Sherrington's Law (Chornell et al., 2010). Perhaps the excess tension of the oblique muscles activates a similar relationship with the rectus muscles during near-point stress.

10.2.3   THE SYNCHRONIZATION OF THE TWO DUAL RELATIONSHIPS IN THE MYOPIC EYE

The third theory is on the synchronization of the two dual relationships of the myopic eye. The first and second myopic relationships are also related to each other. The synchronization of the lens and eyeball can be expressed as follows: the tendency for the crystalline lens to bulge can also cause the eye to elongate.

The third part of the Standard Drill presupposes that such a condition exists. In the second part of the drill, the eyeball retracted a bit more. The crystalline lens needs to readjust for distant focusing by becoming flatter given the renewed shape of the eyeball.

During the onset of myopia, the lens bulges first to induce mild myopia. Then the eyeball becomes elongated next as the refractive error progresses to moderate myopia. The outcome from near-point stress exemplifies the relationship. Initially, the crystalline lens would bulge independent of a change in shape of the eyeball according to the theory of Helmholtz. As the lens reaches its maximum bulged shape and as the patient continues to maintain the object of regard at the nearpoint, the eye would start to elongate to alleviate the stress. The eyeball adapts to the needs of the lens as myopia sets in.

The oblique muscles do not just rotate or turn the eye, but they also orchestrate the function of the rectus muscles and the ciliary muscle for extended near focusing. The two dual relationships are possible due to the common neuropathway: cranial nerve 3 (or C3). The synchronization of the lens and eyeball is activated when the oblique muscles tighten up excessively during near-point stress. It signals the motor cortex that the eyeball needs to assume an elongated shape to alleviate the fatigue imposed on the ciliary muscle during its attempt to maintain the maximum bulged shape of the crystalline lens for prolonged near focusing (Yee, 2014).

The third myopic relationship replaces the neurological relationship between the crystalline lens and the eyeball during development and post-development in the normal or emmetropic eye. Once the first and second myopic relationship is established, those relationships are synchronized.

10.2.4   SYNCHRONIZING THE RIGHT AND LEFT EYE

The fourth theory is on synchronizing the right and left eye. The myopia of one eye impacts the other eye. The fourth myopic relationship can be stated as follows: the excessive tension of the oblique muscle of one eye can also cause the oblique muscles of the other eye to become excessively tense. The binocular visual acuity of a patient with a primary refractive error is usually one line more on the Snellen chart compared with monocular visual acuity. The binocular visual acuity of an anisometropic eye tends to be a line lower than the better eye. It is the prescription of the weaker eye that drags the binocular vision down. It exemplifies the fourth myopic relationship.

The balancing of the right and left eye of an anisometropic patient by applying the Modified Preliminary Drill presupposes that the fourth myopic relationship exists. The treatment relies on the premise that the excess tension of the oblique muscles of the weaker eye is transmitted to the better eye. If that was not the case, the flatter ortho C lens would have an adverse effect on the better eye.

KEYWORDS

- first myopic relationship
- second myopic relationship
- third myopic relationship
- fourth myopic relationship
- oblique muscles
- rectus muscles
- ciliary muscle

PART 2
The Treatment

CHAPTER 11

WHAT NATURAL RELAXATION DRILLS CAN AND CANNOT DO

ABSTRACT

From personal experience and from my participants' experiences, near-sightedness is difficult to treat by relaxation exercises alone. The onset of myopia alters the eye neurologically as well as physiologically. Natural relaxation drills by themselves (such as learning to go about your day without your glasses, palming your eyes, massaging your eyes, etc.) take a long time to restore the proper neurological message.

To complicate matters, myopia can be due to the lens, the cornea, and the eyeball. It is difficult to reduce the elongation of the eyeball or deal with the astigmatic shape of the cornea by natural relaxation alone. The best it can do in the short term is relax the muscle that controls the shape of the crystalline lens: the ciliary muscle. With certain types of refractive errors involving the eyeball and the cornea as well as the crystalline lens, the treatment would be incomplete. I am not saying that it cannot be done. I reiterate, it takes a long time.

Certain types of relaxation exercises can become an extraneous variable when combined with the drills I am proposing. Palming, for example, entices the lens to adopt an occluded neutral shape when the both eyes are occluded. It is different from the open neutral shape it takes on when both eyes are opened when performing the first part of the Preliminary Drill, for example; and it may also be different from the occluded neutral shape it takes on when just one eye is occluded when performing the first part of the Standard Drill. Palming before or after those drills interferes with the outcome.

However, I still encourage participants to palm frequently at any other time—especially when the eye's resistance is high due to a direct induction of stress. Any source responsible for the stress should be addressed first to relieve the spasm before applying any ortho C drills. Without isolating the source, it can revive the stress again to offset the benefit from the treatment. (The chapter *Treating the Loss of Depth Perception* elaborates on the topic.)

11.1   THE LIMITATIONS OF NATURAL RELAXATION EXERCISES

The main difficulty with relaxation exercises lies in depending on relaxing the ciliary muscle directly (instead of indirectly) to stimulate the oblique muscle to relax. Even if those muscles are neurologically linked (by cranial nerve 3 or C3); it is easier for the relaxation of the oblique muscles to stimulate the ciliary muscle indirectly to relax. The regulatory role has changed once you became nearsighted. The ciliary muscle is no longer the control center. It is handed over to the oblique muscles.

In the short term, natural relaxation exercises tend to flatten the crystalline lens by relaxing the ciliary muscle directly. The lens will be doing double work. It has to compensate for its own myopic shape as well as the eyeball. The oblique muscles are still tense, and the eye is still locked in an elongated shape. It is easy for fatigue to set in if the lens is frequently utilizing 100% of its flexibility (or close to it). It should only be utilizing around 50%. Since the oblique muscles are still relatively tight, the excess "effort to see" can induce fluctuations. Although you are sure that you see better, a conventional eye exam would not be able to pick it up. The conditions surrounding such an exam would not allow you to apply 100% of the flexibility of the lens.

11.2   IT IS THE WAY THE MEASUREMENTS ARE TAKEN

Mainstream optometry attributes nearsightedness to the axial length of the eyeball instead of the crystalline lens. The conventional definition for nearsightedness states that it is a condition where the eyeball is too long from front to back. A conventional eye exam bypasses the lens. When prescribing glasses or contact lenses, the crystalline lens is considered too unstable to permit proper focus; but by eliminating its function, the proposed model does not represent the natural eye. The crystalline lens plays a vital part in near and distant focusing. It also synchronizes with the eyeball during development and postdevelopment.

The patients' improvement in visual acuity by natural relaxation exercises cannot be verified by a phoropter during a regular eye exam even if they insist that they can see 20/20—because the treatment just targeted the crystalline lens. A conventional eye exam bypasses the flat shape of the crystalline lens by subjecting it to a variety of techniques: "fogging," conducting the test in a dim room (or a totally dark room), and inadvertently subjecting the eye to "instrument myopia." The way the test is conducted causes the lens to assume a neutral bulged shape instead of a flat shape when attempting to make something out in the distance. The examiner ends up measuring just the eyeball which is still myopic.

11.3   THE PROBLEM WITH FOGGING

"Fogging" involves introducing plus lenses of different powers in front of the eye while the subject tries to read an eye chart 20 ft away. The rationale behind "fogging" is to discourage you from making an "effort to see." It is difficult to see through a plus lens. It is prescribed to patients with hyperopia—not myopia. A nearsighted eye needs a minus lens to bring a distant object into focus. The assumption is that when the eye realizes that it cannot overcome a blur image created by a plus lens, it gives up.

The contention is that making an "effort to see" during the exam can induce ciliary muscle tension and interfere with the outcome. By bypassing the lens, it takes on a neutral shape. A lens in its neutral shape is better than the shape it assumes when the patient makes an "effort to see." However, there is the possibility that the "effort to see" can also be excessive with the introduction of a plus lens. The strain may cause the crystalline lens to adopt a myopic shape if the brain thinks the eye is in near focus mode. It may consider a blur image in the distance as something that is blur close-up—as if the eye was subjected to near-point stress. The ciliary muscle may temporarily seize up before the client gives up trying to see better.

11.4   INSTRUMENT MYOPIA

Instrument myopia is a condition where the eye becomes myopic when an instrument is placed over the eye. Any instrument can create the symptom: a microscope, a telescope, or even a phoropter—the optical equipment used to test your vision. The phenomenon is documented, but it was never taken serious. The assumption in optometry is that the neutral shape of the crystalline lens when the eye is occluded is the same as when regarding an object in the distance, but that is not always the case. Some of my participants with high myopia still visit their eye care specialists for follow-up care. During the initial treatment for severe myopia before the rectus muscles totally regained their tension to maintain the improved shape of the eyeball, my colleagues reported that they see worse when tested with a phoropter compared to trial lenses—even when the examination room was well lit.

By simply occluding one eye while trying to make something out in the distance with the other eye, it activates the lenses in both eyes to take on an occluded neutral shape. One of my participants with compound anisometropia and anisometropic amblyopia is very sensitive to instrument myopia. By covering her better eye with the palm of her hand, she can only make out line 2 on the Snellen chart with her weaker eye. By disengaging her palm a few inches away from the better eye, she can see line 3 instead of line 2 with the weaker eye. And by holding her palm 4 or 5 in. away, she can see line 4 instead of line 3 with the weaker eye.

11.5   THE TYPE OF LIGHT MAKES A DIFFERENCE

The patient sees clearer in the presence of natural light when the aperture of the eye becomes smaller to project the focal point closer to the retina. Good lighting, especially a source of natural light, also allows a "focal point draw" to take place. It is the "focal point draw" that stimulates the crystalline lens to "flatten" for the distance. Under dim lighting conditions during a conventional eye exam, there is a lack of a "focal point draw." The aperture opens wider, and comparable to a single reflex camera, objects would appear blurred. Often just the presence of a dim surrounding is enough to bypass the myopic eye's crystalline lens.

11.6   BYPASSING THE LENS CAN CAUSE AN OVERCORRECTION

Ironically, the patients would realize the improvement in their visual acuity due to natural relaxation when they try on the new glasses. Most of them will experience an overcorrection. The prescription was determined under adverse conditions. It bypassed the lens' ability to flatten to bring a distant object into focus. When conditions become normal, the lens participates in bringing a distant object into focus. The focal point will end up behind the retina instead of on the retina because the power of the lens is too high.

11.7   THE NEUTRAL SHAPE OF THE CRYSTALLINE LENS

There is the assumption that when the eye is occluded, the crystalline lens adopts the same shape as when it attempts to focus on an object far away. In the emmetropic eye that assumption is likely the case. In the myopic eye outside the myopic model, the assumption is also likely to be the case due to the higher restriction imposed on the lens by the spasticity of the ciliary muscle. In the mild and moderate myopic eye within the myopic model, it is possible that the lens' open neutral shape during distant focusing is partially flatter than its occluded neutral shape.

Prior to performing the first part of the Preliminary Drill, the lens already flattened out within the limitation imposed by the tension of the oblique muscles for distant focusing. After the first part of the Preliminary Drill flattens the lens further, the focal point is too close to the retina.

In order to stimulate the eyeball to reduce its elongation, the lens' occluded neutral shape needs to flatten out. It is actually the occluded neutral shape that assumes a myopic shape due to the restriction imposed on the ciliary muscle by the tension of the oblique muscles.

When the first part of the Standard Drill flattens the lens' occluded neutral shape for distant focusing, there is still enough room for the eyeball to retract. The focal does not come too close to the retina. The drill simultaneously triggers a reduction in the elongated shape of the eyeball. The eyeball synchronizes with the reduction in the lens' bulged shape due to the common neural pathway. It is the reverse of what occurs during near-point stress. (Refer to the chapter *The Theory Behind the Resistance Tests*.)

11.8   COMBINING OTHER METHODS WITH ORTHO C?

Ortho C should not be combined with some other types of therapies such as ortho K and plus lens therapy (and all variations of it). They do not mix with ortho C. You cannot perform ortho K, for example, after maximizing the patient's improvement in vision by means of ortho C. Ortho K will erase the benefits gained from ortho C. (For more information, refer to the chapter *How It Reverses Nearsightedness*.)

11.9   CERTAIN NATURAL RELAXATION DRILLS CAN BECOME AN EXTRANEOUS VARIABLE

Do not combine natural relaxation drills with ortho C. Not all relaxation techniques can mix with ortho C. During the drill, the intention is to reset the proper neurological message. Adding a natural relaxation drill to the steps may introduce an extraneous variable. It can neurologically affect the outcome of the drill.

I had one participant with midrange myopia who was very receptive to ortho C. She improved her visual acuity from line 5 to line 9 over the years by performing the Standard Drill. If she palmed her eyes after the drill, however, she would see a bit worse. The relaxation gained from a "contact lens draw" can linger for a few minutes more after the drill. I told her to allow half an hour to an hour for the muscles to stabilize before attempting any relaxation exercises.

She also cannot palm her eyes during the drill. Covering both eyes is comparable to inducing instrument myopia. It causes the occluded neutral shape of the lens to bulge. It can offset the shape of the lens which was just flattened during the first part of the drill but was not given a chance to retain that shape. She also cannot perform it just before the drill. By covering both eyes, the occluded neutral shape of the lens seems to bulge more than the occluded neutral shape it assumes by covering just one eye in the first part of the drill. If the lens bulges more, it does not flatten out as much after the drill.

I would still encourage her to palm now and then as a separate drill whenever she feels that fatigue is about to set in. It should be performed for a few minutes or longer before engaging in extensive reading, working in front of a computer monitor all day, or after extensive work looking at something far away such as copying notes from the blackboard.

11.10   DEMONSTRATING THE LIMITATION OF NATURAL RELAXATION EXERCISES

I can simulate the phenomenon created by natural relaxation exercises by just relaxing the ciliary muscle of a moderate myopic eye with an ortho C lens (which only reverses the myopic shape of the crystalline lens). If you have moderate myopia, and you just perform the first part of the Preliminary Drill, you would experience fluctuations. The first part of the drill is similar to the Wearing Sequence Test. It just attends to the ciliary muscle—and thus the crystalline lens. The Preliminary Drill was mainly designed to treat anisometropia where the ciliary muscle is thicker than usual in the better eye. The crystalline lens is affected in a different way. The lens bulges more in the weaker eye than in the better eye, but the ciliary muscle thickness is equal in both eyes.

By just relaxing the oblique muscles when both eyes are opened, the "contact lens draw" would not stimulate the occluded neutral shape of the lens. Similar to the effect of just relying on natural relaxation exercises, you would see better during the daytime under natural outdoor lighting. Under dim indoor lighting conditions, you would see a bit blur because the aperture of the eye opens wider. It is comparable to an eye exam conducted in a dim room. It bypasses the crystalline lens.

11.11   DEMONSTRATING THE IMPACT OF AN EYE EXAM

11.11.1   AN EYE TREATED BY NATURAL RELAXATION IN THE SHORT TERM

Liberman (1995) noticed the discrepancy between what he knows he can see and what the instruments are telling him. He was able to improve his vision by natural means; but when he tested his vision on the test instruments, it did not register any improvement. He suspected that the problem may lie in the way a conventional test was conducted. In his book, *Take Off Your Glasses and See,* he wrote:

"A month later I seemed to be seeing even more clearly, but when I retested myself, I was surprised to discover no change in my prescription. This was really confusing, because I firmly believed that the only way to show that my vision was improving was to require a weaker prescription.

Even more puzzling was that it seemed my vision had actually deteriorated during the eye exam. What was going on? I began to wonder whether the test conditions could have created a state of physiological stress that had reduced my ability to see clearly."

"Although my prescription wasn't weakening, I continued to increase the time until I was spending the whole day without glasses. I wasn't seeing 20/20, but I could see well enough to know if my patients were reading the eye chart correctly. However, I just didn't know what to make of the experiment at this point. The test instruments were telling me not to believe my own eyes. Everything I had been taught said that I couldn't possibly be seeing better and still have the same old prescription, and yet I was. The contradiction between my beliefs and my actual experience seemed impossible to resolve. I didn't know that what I was about to discover would radically alter all my core beliefs, and not just about vision."

11.11.2   AN EYE TREATED BY ORTHO C IN THE SHORT TERM

A participant had anisometropia and high astigmatism. He was going through the application process for law enforcement, and his vision test was coming up in a couple of weeks. The following was his present prescription: OD −1.00–1.50 × 60 and OS −2.00–0.50 × 170. An optometrist would sign off on the form only when he meets the requirement. Thus, he had to go through a conventional eye exam.

He has anisometropia and high astigmatism. His astigmatism made it more difficult to close the gap in prescription between the right and left eye. High astigmatism is the main challenge facing proponents of natural relaxation exercises. I have a participant who managed to reduce her myopia significantly over a period of 10 years, but her high astigmatism remained the same.

To add to the difficulty, I only had time to treat him for a week. I decided to apply the Modified Preliminary Drill. There was no time to resort to the Preliminary Drill first. In his case, it was not necessary. It would not have worked since his cylinder is more than 100% of the sphere in the better eye. He directly performed the Modified Preliminary Drill three times on different days before his eye exam. He informed me later that he passed the exam. The results were as follows: OD 20/25 and OS 20/50.

The RCMP (Royal Canadian Mounted Police) requires 20/40 in one eye. Going by his initial prescription, it would have been difficult for him to pass the test. If you look at the conversion chart from Snellen reading measurements to diopters in the *Addendum*, a visual acuity of 20/40 requires a prescription of −0.75 D for his right eye. His prescription was −1.00–1.50 × 60. Not only was his sphere higher (−1.00 D), he also had astigmatism of −1.50 D. (Refer to the chapters *The Theory Behind the Modified Preliminary Drill*, *Treating Anisometropia*, and *Treating Astigmatism* for more information.)

KEYWORDS

- palming
- axial length
- fogging
- instrument myopia
- lens' open neutral shape
- lens' occluded neutral shape
- plus lens therapy

CHAPTER 12

DESIGNING THE LENS

ABSTRACT

The following are the main differences between a flexible ortho C lens and a conventional hard contact lens (or rigid gas permeable lens):

- There is no prescription.
- It is slightly flatter (or less curved) than the curvature of your cornea. (A generic rigid gas permeable lens is already designed to be slightly flatter than the flat meridian of the cornea for a better fit.)
- It is slightly thinner and thus more flexible. (It is still within the thickness specifications proposed by Stein et al. (2002). It is classified as a thin design.)

There are two kinds of contact lens available on the market: soft and hard. If you are familiar with wearing a soft contact lens, it is easier to adapt to an ortho C lens. If your client is unfamiliar with wearing a contact lens, it will probably take a few applications before the eye can adapt to the lens I am recommending. Although an ortho C lens is still referred to as a "hard" or rigid gas permeable lens (RGP lens), it is more flexible. When you hold an ortho C lens by the edge between your thumb and forefinger and gently squeeze it, it will flex a bit. A typical hard contact lens is very stiff.

Although the lens has no prescription, it is not a generic design. It must specifically address the different ranges of myopia—whether it is mild, moderate, midrange, or severe myopia. In this publication, we are just dealing with the mild and moderate range.

The flatness of the lens is generally equal to the absolute value (ignoring the minus sign) of your client's prescription as outlined in the chapter *Specifications*. An ortho C lens is slightly flatter than the curvature of the cornea, but it is not as flat as an orthokeratology (ortho K) lens.

Wearing a flatter lens is not unusual. A conventional RGP lens is already designed to be flatter than the cornea in order to achieve a better fit.

12.1   THE HYPOTHESIS ON THE TREATMENT

12.1.1   THE HYPOTHESIS

When a "contact lens draw" is combined with a "focal point draw," it triggers a reversal in myopia by "loosening" the oblique muscles. Once the shapes of the lens and eyeball are not restricted by the tension of the oblique muscles, the brain considers the eye to be emmetropic. It stimulates the eye neurologically to correct itself. The process is the reverse of near-point stress.

12.1.2   THE DESIGN BASED ON THE HYPOTHESIS

The design of the lens must loosen the oblique muscles sufficiently to release the restriction imposed on how much the ciliary muscle can relax in order for the crystalline lens to flatten for distant focusing. The design of the lens must also loosen the oblique muscles sufficiently to allow the rectus muscles to tighten up in order for the eye to reduce its elongation. The responsiveness to the treatment relies on the premise that the myopic eye falls within the myopic model.

12.2   THE IMPORTANCE OF REMOVING THE PRESCRIPTION

An important feature of an ortho C lens is that it is a plain or "plano" lens, as it is sometimes referred to in optometry parlance. Without removing the prescription, the lens would not produce the proper stimulation even if it meets all the other specifications.

Adding a prescription to the lens would interfere with a "focal point draw." The focal point would be on the retina instead of being slightly in front of it when attempting to bring something in the distance into focus. The longer focal length locks in the crystalline lens and sclera to their myopic shape.

With a plain lens, there is the absence of a fixed focal length to restrict any possible improvement. Its elimination is one of the main reasons why a "focal point draw" is possible. The focal point of a mild or moderate myopic eye would be slightly in front of the retina. The gap allows a "focal point draw" to take place. An object must be slightly blur (by being slightly in front of the retina) before the "contact lens draw" can generate a "focal point draw." (Refer to the chapter *How It Reverses Nearsightedness* for more information.)

12.3   ITS FLATNESS

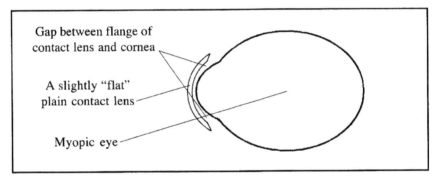

FIGURE 12.1   An ortho C lens slightly flatter than the cornea.

The ortho C lens' flatness makes a "contact lens draw" possible. Its flatness factor refers to the difference between the curvature of the contact lens and the curvature of the cornea. An ortho C lens is said to be "flatter" than the cornea because it is less curved as illustrated in Figure 12.1. (If it was more curved, it would be "steeper.") As the lens becomes flatter, the gap between the edge of the contact lens and the cornea becomes wider.

The lens' flatness represents the tension inherited by the oblique muscles—as well as how much the crystalline lens and eyeball deviated from their normal shape (due to that tension). The "contact lens draw" reverses the deviation when the lens flatness "draws" against the cornea to relax the oblique muscles. Thus, the design of the lens has neurological implications. (Refer to the chapter *How It Reverses Nearsightedness* for more information on the "contact lens draw.")

If you have mild or moderate myopia, you cannot wear a lens designed for severe myopia. Otherwise your vision would be overcorrected. It should only treat the part of the eye that deviated, and the correction has to be within the range of deviation. (Refer to the chapter *Reinstating the Correct Message* for more information.)

The lens' flatness is in relation to the patient's prescription. It must be calculated properly before the "contact lens draw" is correct, and the "contact lens draw" needs to be correct before the "focal point draw" is correct. (Refer to the chapter *The Procedure* for information on calculating the lens' base curve.) Its flatness is equal to the absolute value of the prescription in mild and moderate cases of myopia. The flatness factor is from 0.25 D to 0.75 D for mild myopia and 1.00 D to 1.75 D for moderate myopia. A diopter is a measurement of refractive error. It is also used to represent the curvature of your cornea.

If a contact lens is too flat, it would be easier for the flange of the lens to separate from the meniscus of the contact lens solution and tears. The lens would end up exerting pressure against the cornea instead of wrapping around it. The lens must wrap around the cornea before it can produce a "draw." If the meniscus fails to "draw" it onto the cornea, it may induce ortho K instead of ortho C. Ortho K is designed to flatten the cornea to promote better vision. Ortho K and ortho C do not mix. (More information is given in the chapter *How It Reverses Nearsightedness*.)

The intention of ortho C is not to change the curvature of the cornea but to "draw" against it—like the way a bow would "draw" against the string. The "string" in this case is actually the contact lens solution. When the meniscus "draws" the lens onto the cornea, the reactionary force from the lens pulls against it. The meniscus adheres along the flange of the lens, and it transmits the "draw" onto the cornea. The "draw" does not alter the curvature of the cornea due to its minimum flatness and the short wearing time, but it can still stimulate the muscles of the eye. The cornea behaves like a contact lens and transmits the "draw" onto the sclera.

The meniscus allows a continuous "contact lens draw" of the same magnitude. Although the solution and tears would eventually drain from an ortho C lens, remind the patient to take the lens out before that happens. The optimum period for the stimulation to work effectively is within the first 5 min depending on the flatness of the lens. The flatter the lens, the quicker the solution would drain, and the lens would push against the cornea.

12.4   ITS THICKNESS

An ortho C contact lens is not as thick as a conventional hard prescription contact lens. It is the prescription that makes a generic rigid contact lens thicker. A plus lens is thicker starting from the center, and a minus lens is thicker starting from the edge. An ortho C lens is not strictly a hard contact lens because its thickness is 0.15 mm as oppose to the standard thickness of 0.17 or 0.18 mm for a plain RGP lens. An ortho C lens is actually a flexible lens.

It is flexible enough to wrap around the cornea instead of "pushing" against it. It conforms to the contour of the cornea when the meniscus of the contact lens solution pulls the lens towards the cornea to reduce the gap between the flange of the contact lens and the cornea as in Figure 12.1. The lens then produces a reactionary "draw."

The lens cannot be too flexible. A lens which is very thin will not work. If it is less than 0.14 mm thick, it would not produce an adequate reactionary "draw." I do not resort to a lens 0.14-mm thick, even though it still works, because it warps easier. A RGP lens cut 0.15-mm thick will last for years when the patient handles it with care—especially if the diameter is 9.2 mm or less. There is no safety issue with a lens cut 0.15-mm thick. It falls within the parameter of what is considered as a thin design (Stein et al., 2002).

A lens with a thickness of 0.16 mm can produce a greater "draw." Although it produces an adequate "draw," there is always the risk that you would end up applying ortho K—depending on the duration of wear. I have applied a 0.16-mm lens to reduce severe corneal astigmatism. I want to produce a "draw" that is intense enough to gradually realign the rectus muscles over time. Then again, it depends on the flatness of the lens.

A lens thicker than 0.16 mm can produce an even greater "draw," but it does not exhibit an adequate "draw." An adequate "draw" is a "draw" which is strong enough to stimulate the muscles of the eye but not so strong that the flange of the lens separates from the meniscus and end up "pushing" against the cornea. The stiffness of a lens thicker than 0.16 mm would tend to depress the cornea instead of wrapping around it. It would be like wearing a lens that is too flat.

When ordering the lenses online for your patient, make sure that you specified its center thickness which is 0.15 mm. There is an entry for the other measurements; but the thickness is not one of the options given. You have to emphasize the thickness in the space where it allows you to give your comments. If you order from a lab instead, it ensures that the thickness is correct. Even if the other specifications of the lenses are correct, the lens would not produce the proper "draw" if its thickness is incorrect.

12.5   ITS DIAMETER

The diameter of an ortho C lens is 9.20 or 9.50 mm. It can be slightly larger than 9.50 mm and still produce an adequate "draw." According to conventional fitting, the actual diameter depends on the opening of your client's lids. I generally select a diameter of 9.20 mm. A lens of this diameter is compatible for teens as well as adults, and it is applicable for people with narrow as well as normal lids opening. In the odd case where a 9.20 mm is too large due to a narrow lids opening, I would reduce it to 9.0 mm. A 9.20-mm lens offers more durability. It extends the life of the lens. I had clients using the same lens with that diameter for over a decade. There is less flexing, but there is enough flexure to produce a "contact lens draw." It also allows a better chance for the lens to be cut within tolerance given a thickness of 0.15 mm compared to a lens with a larger diameter.

A larger diameter, such as a 10.0-mm lens, can still allow an adequate "draw," but the lens can bind to the cornea. The larger diameter (given the same radius) means that more surface area comes into contact with the cornea; there would be less gap between the flange of the lens and the cornea because its curvature would follow the contour of the cornea. It is more likely to be sucked-on when air is pushed out by rubbing the eye with the lens on or by blinking a lot if your client has tight lids. By pushing against the lens, it creates a suction. (Refer to the *Addendum* on how to remove a sucked-on lens.)

If a 9.50-mm lens still sticks slightly, you may have to resort to a smaller diameter. If your client has dry eyes, the drop of solution that you would place on the lens before insertion would help. (You need to apply a drop before insertion anyway to enable a "contact lens draw".) If necessary, before removal, wet the head of the plunger with contact lens solution. This lubricates the cornea again once the plunger touches the contact lens. I have lots of patients with dry eyes who cannot wear conventional contact lenses, but they have no problem with the ortho C lenses.

By reducing the diameter, (given the same radius), there is more gap between the flange of the lens and the cornea. It allows more tears to filter in. You reduce the chance of adhesion by decreasing the amount of surface that comes into contact with the cornea (while still maintaining an adequate "draw").

12.6   TYPE OF MATERIAL

The material should be "flexible" enough to induce a "drawing" effect. I had worked with different materials and found that the Boston EO lens (or equivalent) works best. The Boston XO lens is too soft, and Boston ES is too stiff. The Boston EO lens is firm enough to allow it to be 0.15-mm thick and still generates a maximum "draw" up to a flatness of 2.00 D. I had success with other types of materials which are more firm (or less porous, and thus less flexible), but they are too stiff to allow an adequate "draw" if the flatness is over 1.0 D.

12.7   AN ORTHO C LENS POSES LESS RISK THAN A CONVENTIONAL CONTACT LENS

An ortho C lens has no prescription. Considering that feature by itself makes it less risky than a conventional hard contact lens which has a prescription. The fixed focal length of a conventional contact lens constricts the ciliary muscle (and eventually the oblique muscles), and it contributes to progressive myopia. An ortho C lens is porous enough to be flexible instead of rigid. It is not so flexible that you can fold it until the edge meets as you could with a soft lens, but it is flexible enough to allow it to wrap around the cornea instead of depressing it. The few minutes the patient has the lenses on reduces eye infection compared to conventional contact lens wear.

The concept of wearing a contact lens slightly flatter than the curvature of the cornea is not a revolutionary idea. It is a common practice for a conventional rigid prescription lens to be a bit flatter. The intention is to improve the fit of the lens on one of the meridian—the "flatter K." So you may already have a flat pair of lenses if you are presently wearing RGP lenses. It is just that you may not be aware of it. An ortho C lens is even less flat than a conventional RGP lens. The latter is flatter than the "flatter k" while the former is flatter than the "mid k"—the average between the steeper and flatter k. There is a big difference between my lens and an ortho K lens. An ortho K lens, as described in more detail in the next chapter, is much flatter.

Although wearing an ortho C lens poses less risk compared to a regular contact lens, keep in mind that it is for therapeutic use only. It is not to be worn as a visual aid—like a normal hard or soft contact lens. You would never wear it like an ortho K lens because it is not "flat" enough. Besides, you cannot combine ortho C with ortho K since ortho K is an extraneous variable.

KEYWORDS

- **lens' flatness**
- **lens' steepness**
- **contact lens draw**
- **focal point draw**
- **lens' thickness**
- **lens' diameter**

CHAPTER 13

HOW IT REVERSES
NEARSIGHTEDNESS

ABSTRACT

A contact lens is slightly flatter than the cornea. It produces a contact lens draw when the meniscus from the contact lens solution pulls the edge of the lens inward. The reactionary force pulls outwards against the cornea. The cornea acts like a rigid contact lens and draws outwards on the sclera. The eyeball tends to become less elongated and thicker around the middle to reduce the strangle hold of the oblique muscles around that part of the eye. When the brain interprets the eye to be in distant focus mode (instead of near focus mode when the oblique muscles were tense), the "focal point draw" then flattens the crystalline lens and eyeball once the motor cortex sends the proper message to the ciliary and rectus muscles.

The power of the prescription determines the flatness of the contact lens, and its flatness determines its "draw." A "contact lens draw" "loosens" the tension of the oblique muscles to allow a "focal point draw." The flatness must be correct before it neutralizes the mild or moderate myopia. Ortho C attends to the following relationship: there is a correlation between the prescription expressed in diopters and the lens' equivalent flatness—also expressed in diopters. The calculation for the flatness factor is given in the chapter *The Procedure*.

If your prescription is -1.25 D for both eyes, then the flatness factor is 1.25 D. You would expect the cornea to flatten out or become less steep by 1.25 D, but it does not. The curvature remains the same to allow a constant draw of 1.25 D to "loosen" the oblique muscles when the "draw" from the lens is transmitted to the cornea. The cornea becomes an extension of the contact lens and "draws" against the eye to make it wider from top to bottom and side to side. Theoretically, the oblique muscles' tightness decreases by 1.25 D.

The ortho C lens does not actually reverse your nearsightedness. It is the motor cortex responding to the correct neurosensory message: a blur image in the distance and a more relaxed set of oblique muscles when you look at something far away. The brain initiates the proper neuromotor message to the ciliary muscle and rectus muscles when it interprets the decrease in tension as an eye that is in distant focus mode.

13.1   DIFFERENCE BETWEEN ORTHO C AND ORTHO K

Ortho C is not the same as an existing method on the market known as orthokeratology (or ortho K). Ortho C is the opposite of ortho K. Ortho K pushes instead of "drawing" on the cornea to promote an improvement in vision. I selected ortho K as a contrast to the treatment I am proposing to help you realize the implications of wearing an ortho C lens. Once you know, for example, about the limitations and drawbacks of ortho K, you will realize the extent what ortho C can do.

Suppose you have severe myopia, and the eyeball as well as the crystalline lens assumed a myopic shape. Ortho K attempts to improve your visual acuity by flattening the cornea with a special rigid gas-permeable contact lens. The intention is to alter the curvature of the cornea with a flat lens so that it assumes the same curvature as the contact lens. The modified cornea, similar to a minus lens, promotes an improvement in vision by diverging the rays of light from a distant image to bring its focal point closer to the retina. You have to wear those lenses every night while you are asleep. When you would take them off in the morning, you would see clearer if the cornea retains the change in curvature.

Your vision can become myopic again if you miss wearing them for a day or two. Ortho C offers a more flexible schedule. If you missed wearing the lens for a few days according to a specific schedule, it is no big deal; you just continue the wearing schedule the following day. Similar to forgetting to go to the gym on the day that you planned to go, it does not mean that you would gain back the excess weight you shed.

In a former variation of ortho K, you would wear the lenses during the day. The design of the lens includes a reduced prescription. The flatness of the lens makes up for the difference by molding the cornea to conform to its flatness. The intention is to improve your vision by an amount dictated by the flatness of the lens in order to project the focal point closer to the retina for distant focusing. Then a flatter lens and a lower prescription would be assigned to the next lens. After your cornea conforms to the shape of that lens, another flatter lens is assigned to flatten your cornea a little more, and your prescription would be reduced a bit more, and so on, until 20/20 vision is achieved. It is comparable to orthodontics where poorly aligned teeth are slowly and gradually moved into a better position when the braces gradually force them into a predetermined shape. The lack of success with the technique lies in the difficult to incrementally change the cornea curvature.

Although an ortho C lens is also flatter than the curvature of your cornea, an ortho K lens is much flatter than an ortho C lens' maximum flatness for moderate myopia which is 1.75 D. The maximum flatness for an overnight ortho K lens can be up to 6.00 D. The flattened cornea has to compensate for the myopic shape of the eyeball as well as the crystalline lens. An ortho K lens is also thicker. The extra flatness and thickness ensure that when the lens pushes against the cornea, the cornea will adopt the new shape. The improvement is due to the change in the curvature of the cornea. With ortho C, the improvement in visual acuity is not due to the change in the shape of the cornea. It is the result of altering the curvature of both the crystalline lens and the eyeball.

The problem with ortho K is that regardless of how often and how long you attempt to flatten the cornea, there is always the tendency for it to creep back to its former myopic shape. Its shape is not regulated by any muscle. The shape of the lens and eyeball, on the other hand, is determined by the intraocular and extraocular muscles. By applying ortho C to reestablish the proper neurological control of those muscles, it offers your vision more stability.

13.2   THE THEORY ON THE TREATMENT

Prior to ortho C, the motor cortex ignores the myopee's perception of a distant object even though the subject knows that it is far away. Due to the tension of the oblique muscles, the brain interprets the eye to be in near focus mode. It bypasses the neurosensory message of a blur distant object. When a "contact lens draw" "loosens" the oblique muscles' grip around the eyeball, the motor cortex will then take the subject's depth perception of a distant image into account. It recognizes that the eye is in distant focus mode.

The motor cortex reinstates the correct neuromuscular message to allow distant objects to come into focus. A "focal point draw" reverses the bulged shape of the crystalline lens when the correct neuromotor message relaxes the ciliary muscle for distant focusing. It simultaneously reverses the elongated eyeball when the correct neuromotor message tightens the rectus muscles for distant focusing. The myopic crystalline lens must flatten first before the myopic eyeball can retract.

13.2.1   THE DRAWING FORCE

The ortho C lens is slightly flatter than the cornea. It is flexible enough to wrap around the cornea. The cornea should collapse the contact lens—not the other way around. If the contact lens depresses the cornea, then the lens is too thick, or too flat, or both. The outcome would then resemble ortho K instead of ortho C.

The patient must apply a drop of contact lens solution onto the lens before insertion. The lens does not actually rest on the cornea but on a layer of contact lens solution. The solution acts as an artificial cornea. Most corneas exhibit an astigmatic shape due to the difference in the horizontal and vertical curvature. The contact lens liquid fills in the uneven areas and permits the lens to adhere to it evenly.

The contact lens is slightly flatter than the cornea, so there is a gap between the lens and the cornea. The meniscus pulls the portion of the lens near the flange inwards until it bends like a bow to reduce the gap between the contact lens and the corner. The meniscus acts like the string of a bow to maintain the shape of the lens. When the lens flexes inward to meet the cornea, it is not the same as holding it between the index finger and thumb and squeezing it slightly. The pressure only bends certain parts of the lens. A fluid, on the other hand, comes into contact with the lens as a whole. When a fluid pulls on the lens, it does not bend at a specific meridian but all along the perimeter of the lens.

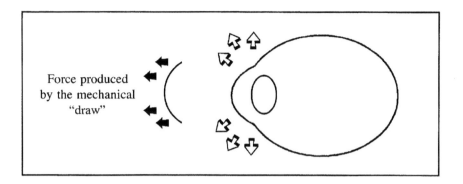

The lens produces a reactionary force by "drawing" outward against the inward suction as it strives to return back to its original curvature. The "contact lens draw" is not like the suction produced by a plunger. When you pull on a plunger, the suction is stronger at the center of the lens, and it dissipates in the direction towards the edge. The "contact lens draw" is more powerful along the edge of the lens, and it dissipates in the direction towards the center of the lens, but it is not so strong that it breaks the meniscus. The outward "draw" is even all around the perimeter of the lens and is equally transmitted by the meniscus to the cornea.

13.2.2 IT LOWERS THE RESISTANCE OF THE OBLIQUE MUSCLES

A "contact lens draw" does not actually spread out the cornea, but it creates the *tendency* to do so. The cornea in turn transmits the "draw" to the eyeball. The cornea acts like a rigid ortho C contact lens and draws on the sclera outwards in the direction of the arrows. The direction of the pull of the cornea is slightly more outwards compared to the pull of the contact lens because the curvature of the cornea is steeper than the contact lens. It is the outward "draw" of the cornea that "loosens" the oblique muscles.

13.3 THE FOCAL POINT DRAW

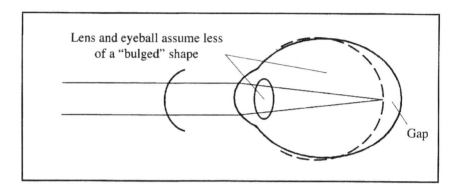

The gap between the focal point of a distant object and the retina allows a "focal point draw." The gap is produced by the myopic shape of the crystalline lens and eyeball which are too long from front to back. When the focal point is at a certain distance from the retina, it tends to stimulate the lens to "shift" (to bring the focal point closer to the retina) or the eyeball to "shift" (to bring the retina closer to the focal point).

13.3.1 A FOCAL POINT DRAW ALONE

The projection of a focal point by itself cannot stimulate the curvature of the crystalline lens or eyeball to change to bring a distant image into focus. Otherwise an ortho C lens is not required to relax the oblique muscles. All you would need is to have a weaker minus lens projecting a focal point within a reasonable distance in front of the retina. But it is difficult for a "focal point draw" by itself to cause a change in visual acuity because the oblique muscles are still too tight.

Most of the researches done on treating nearsightedness are actually an application of a "focal point draw" without the assistance of a "contact lens draw"—such as wearing weaker glasses to improve one's vision. Any positive results are not as quick or as pronounced as ortho C due to the absence of a "contact lens draw." Some researchers encountered the problem of an "effort to see" among the participants and had to discontinue the research when such an effort adds to the existing tension to make their vision worse. When the oblique muscles are not sufficiently "loosened," the visual cortex still regards the eye to be in near focus mode.

13.3.2 A CONTACT LENS DRAW ALONE

A "contact lens draw" alone cannot improve your visual acuity. It only produces a mechanical "draw." By itself, it cannot alter the curvature of the crystalline lens or eyeball. You can prove that by closing your eyes while wearing the lenses. You will not experience any visual improvement when you take them off. A "shift" did not take place. This simple experiment demonstrates that a change in the curvature of the crystalline lens or eyeball can only be produced when a mechanical "draw" combines with a "focal point draw" to reverse the myopic eye neurologically.

13.4 COMBINING THE TWO TYPES OF DRAW

When you wear an ortho C lens, you do not just experience the influence of a "contact lens draw" or a "focal point draw." Instead, you benefit from their combined contribution which is different from what each has to offer. It is like cooking. When you combine different ingredients, you end up with a different flavor—and a different dish.

A "contact lens draw" produces the tendency for the eye to become longer from top to bottom and from side to side (when viewed from the front) and shorter from front to back (when viewed from the side). The movement slightly "loosens" the oblique muscles. The reduction in tension eases the strangle hold those muscles have around the center of the eyeball. The brain interprets the eye to be in distant focus mode instead of near focus mode. When a "focal point draw" combines with a "contact lens draw," the motor cortex generates the proper neuromuscular message to "stretch" the oblique muscles (whereas the "contact lens draw" initially "loosens" it). The oblique muscles act as a relay switch to channel the modified message to the ciliary and rectus muscles to orchestrate the change in distant focusing (Yee, 2011).

The correct neuromuscular message relaxes the ciliary muscle to allow the crystalline lens to flatten. It removes the restriction placed on the ciliary muscle to limit how much the crystalline lens can flatten. It also tightens the rectus muscles to allow the eyeball to retract. The "stretching" of the oblique muscles allowed sufficient room for the eye to "shift." The reversal of the first and second myopic relationships suggests that the oblique muscles adopted a regulatory role once the eye became myopic. (Refer to the chapter *Neurological Implications* for more information on the first and second myopic relationships.)

13.5   INCREASE IN RETENTION

13.5.1   *NOT RESHAPING THE LENS OR SCLERA DIRECTLY*

The retention of the improved shape of the lens and sclera for distant focusing is longer than ortho K because the "contact lens draw" stimulates the intraocular and extraocular muscles. It did not attempt to reverse the curvature of the crystalline lens or eyeball directly but indirectly—by stimulating the muscles that control them. Your improved visual acuity after being treated by ortho K is shorter because the shape of the cornea is not controlled by any muscle. (Refer to the chapter *The Theory Behind the Standard Drill* for other reasons why there is an increase in retention.)

13.5.2   *ATTENDING TO BOTH THE LENS AND THE EYEBALL*

By resetting the interrelationship of the intraocular and extraocular muscles, it promotes the increase in retention. You are not improving just the shape of the lens or just the shape of the eyeball. You are attending to both the lens and eyeball because the intraocular and extraocular muscles were affected when the eye became myopic. If you just improved the shape of the crystalline lens in moderate myopia, for example, the ciliary muscle would have to perform more work to bring a distant object into focus. The extra "effort to see" contributes to an increase in fluctuation.

13.6   ADHERING TO THE SAME FLATNESS FACTOR AFTERWARDS

13.6.1   *CONVENTIONAL APPLICATION*

Although there is an improvement in visual acuity, you still adhere to the same "contact lens draw" to relax the oblique muscles when it is time to perform the drill again according to the wearing schedule. It was based on the patient's initial prescription. It is not necessary to change the lens' base curve after the visual acuity improves. If your patient's prescription was −1.50 D, and you improved the visual acuity to −0.25 D, the patient would still retain the same lens with a flatness factor of 1.50 D. You do not change it to 0.25 D. Performing the drill with a lens that has a lower flatness factor will reduce the visual acuity even after one application.

The flatness factor of 1.50 D represents the amount of tension that needs to be subtracted once a "contact lens draw" activates a "focal point draw." It is in reference to the original prescription when the eye was −1.50 D. The patient requires a flatness factor of 1.50 to establish emmetropia. As the prescription changed to −0.25 D, for example, the lens does not subtract another −1.50 D of tension when you wear it again and perform the necessary drill. The lens would not overcorrect the myopic eye. The base curve of 1.50 D represents the curvature of the emmetropic eye. The outcome of −0.25 D is a residual tension after initially applying a "contact lens draw" of 1.50 D.

13.6.2   AN EXCEPTION

There is an exception to basing the flatness factor on the initial prescription. If your patient had laser surgery and if the visual acuity regressed by −0.50 D, for example, you would not resort to the original prescription. Suppose the original prescription was −3.00 D. An adjustment was already made by shaving off the cornea by that amount to make it flatter. The oblique muscles' excessive tension was accounted for. It became the norm to establish equilibrium. A regression of −0.50 D would be treated as a new prescription. The tension of the oblique muscles increased by 0.50 D above the norm. You would design a lens with a base curve 0.50 D flatter than mid K to offset the increase. Such a lens produces a "contact lens draw" of 0.50 D. If you went by the original prescription, the "draw" on the cornea is too high. Such a flatness factor would produce a total "draw" of 3.50 D to offset the present deviation of −0.50 D.

KEYWORDS

- ortho C
- ortho K
- rigid gas-permeable contact lens
- motor cortex
- meniscus
- contact lens draw
- focal point draw

CHAPTER 14

THE PROCEDURE

ABSTRACT

At first glance, it may seem that there are a lot of details. I also included information on acquiring the right tools and lens design as well as dealing with the different types of refractive errors you may encounter.

Pay particular attention to the Wearing Sequence Test. The patient must wear the lens and perform the drill in the correct sequence if the lenses are worn one at a time. If both lenses are worn together, you still need to know which eye performs the drill first. It is straightforward when dealing with a primary refractive error and most types of secondary refractive errors. The exception is when you are dealing with compound anisometropia and anisometropic amblyopia. The wearing sequence is reversed.

The information in this chapter provides the context for the drills given in the chapter *What to Do*. I wrote the following procedure for other professionals as well as the eye care specialist. Thus, I clarified certain terminology and elaborated on some of the steps. Performing the treatment is easier than you think once the preparations are in place. Refer to the examples in the chapter *Case Examples* as a guide.

14.1 MATERIALS, MEASUREMENTS, AND INSTRUCTIONS

The following are some preparations you need to make:

For test purposes, rely on trial lenses instead of a phoropter to avoid the possibility of inducing instrument myopia. You want the crystalline lens to participate in the visual acuity test to help determine the weaker eye in Step 6 if the prescription of both eyes is the same or close to being the same. The information is necessary to establish the wearing sequence in Step 7. The correct wearing sequence for the specific drill synchronizes the right and left eye.

If you do not have any trial lenses and if you do not want to purchase a complete set (which consists of a frame and different lenses in the plus and minus ranges), purchase the following pairs of glasses online: −0.25 D, −0.50 D, −0.75 D, and −1.00 D. Although the pupil distance (PD) measurement is different for different patients, order the glasses with an average range of 60 mm. A few millimeters off compared with your patient's actual PD is okay with a low prescription. These glasses can also serve as your inventory. Any client with a "partial resistance" may need a pair within that range.

You need a Snellen chart calibrated for 10 ft. It is more practical in a standard size office than a 20-ft eye chart. You need a 10-ft chart anyway when the patient performs the Snellen Chart Drill. The size of the letters is smaller. The big E, for example, is 1.75 in. high. A chart is included in this book. When you copy it, measure the big E to ensure that the height is correct. If it is, then the other letters are in the proper proportion.

You also need a rigid gas permeable (RGP) lens remover to remove the contact lens. You can purchase some from an optical supplier, an optical outlet, from eBay, or Amazon.com. Refer to the *Addendum* on how to apply a plunger. The slight flexibility of the lens allows the meniscus to reduce the gap between the perimeter of the lens and the cornea. It is difficult to wedge the lids into the gap to remove the lens in the conventional manner. I included in the *Addendum* an explanation on the conventional way to remove the lens and on emergency removal in case the client loses the plunger. You should give the client an extra plunger as a precaution.

Have a magnifying glass and penlight handy in case you need them during a follow-up. Refer to the *Addendum* for information on purchasing the proper contact lens solution for RGP lenses—not for soft contact lenses. Have several bottles ready. Have a fair size mirror that allows the patient to adjust the angle. Position it at about 30° from the table to allow the patient to bend down when inserting the lens; otherwise, the solution may drain before the lens is on the cornea. There should be enough solution between the lens and cornea to create a uniform "contact lens draw." For removal, you need to have the mirror in an upright position. It allows the patient to see the rim easier and to find the lens if it inadvertently shifted off-center.

You need certain measurements from the patient: the latest prescription (within a year) and a keratometer reading (k reading). If you do not have a keratometer, your patient can obtain a k reading from an eye care specialist at a retail outlet such as Costco or Walmart or from a private optometrist (although the latter tends to charge more). (Refer to the *Addendum* for more information on what a k reading entails.)

Instruct the client on contact lens removal and insertion, how to apply the plunger, and cleaning the lenses. Emphasize the importance of applying a drop of contact lens solution onto the lens before insertion. You may also want to explain some of the relaxation, swinging, and stretching exercises. (Refer to the *Addendum* for information on those topics.)

14.2 STEP 1

14.2.1 CHECK THE PATIENT'S HISTORY

Ask about the patient's medical and ocular history to rule out any extraneous variables. Check the date of the prescription. It should be within a year to ensure that it is still valid. Consider the age of the patient. Inquire when the refractive error set in. I had a participant, for example, who was 15 years of age. Her prescription was −1.00 D. She hardly wore her glasses. Her resistance should have been low, but she was not that responsive to ortho C. I found that her myopia started several years ago. If the development of her eye was ongoing during that period, it may have accounted for her partial resistance.

Determine any other offsetting variables that may interfere with ortho C. Familiarize yourself with the list of negative variable from the chapter *Extraneous Variables* so that you can relate the information to your patient. Determine any bad habits that may promote an increase in "effort to see." It may be difficult to break the habit immediately. Remind your client that any of them can linger after the treatment, and they have to be dealt with separately. An opposite behavior requires a certain amount of repetition—about 66 times. (Refer to the chapter *The Effort to See* for more information.)

14.3 STEP 2

14.3.1 CHECK THE VISUAL ACUITY PRIOR TO PERFORMING ANY DRILLS

14.3.1.1 PRIOR TO PERFORMING THE DRILL

Perform a Visual Acuity Test with an eye chart calibrated for 10 ft instead of 20 ft to minimize any excessive "effort to see." The increase in distance may trigger mental strain. At 10 ft away, the rays of light are slightly divergent; but it is negligible. Hang the chart by a source of natural light 10 ft away. If you do not have access to a window that allows natural lighting, then hang the chart in adequate lighting. The room should be well lit so that minor changes in visual acuity would be noticeable. Line 8 is the 20/20 line. It represents normal visual acuity during the day since you are conducting the test in adequate light. If the patient can read line 9 or 10, it represents normal visual acuity at night.

If the patient has mild myopia, set the benchmark by taking a visual acuity test with the naked eye if the prescription is −0.50 D or −0.75 D. You may want to decline treating anyone with −0.25 D in both eyes by ortho C. (Refer to the section *Calculate the Base Curve* for more information.) If the patient's prescription is in the moderate range from −1.00 D to −1.75D, take a visual acuity test with a pair of −0.50 D or −0.75 D trial lenses as well as with the naked eye. Those results serve as benchmarks. The power is undercorrected by two or three lines on the Snellen chart because you expect the visual acuity of the patient to improve by two or three lines. The pretest and posttest results offer proof to the patient that there is an improvement in visual acuity.

If a pair of glasses was prescribed, check the visual acuity with them on. If the patient cannot see the 20/20 line with the glasses, it is an indication that his visual acuity had deteriorated. So instead of mild myopia, for example, it progressed to moderate myopia. Make sure the patient is not squinting when reading the eye chart. Measure also the naked eye's binocular and monocular visual acuity. (Refer to the *Addendum* for the steps involved in performing and recording a Visual Acuity Test.)

14.3.1.2   AFTER PERFORMING THE DRILL

Perform a visual acuity test after performing the specific drill to determine the before and after result. Prior to performing any drills, the patient may see line 4 with the naked eye, for example, and line 5 with the −0.50 D glasses. After performing the Standard Drill, the patient may see line 7 with the naked eye and line 9 with the −0.50 D glasses. In this case, the eye responds better to the weaker glasses. There is less "effort to see" with the glasses on.

14.3.1.3   MAIN PURPOSE OF A VISUAL ACUITY TEST

The following data summarize why you need a visual acuity test:

- The visual acuity test serves as a benchmark to demonstrate how much the patient's visual acuity has improved after the first application—after wearing the ortho C lenses and performing the specific drill for the first time. The main indicator is the before and after binocular vision results. It is common to see one line less on the Snellen chart with each eye separately compared to both eyes. When occluding one eye, it exposes the occluded neutral myopic shape of both eyes. It is more bulged than the open neutral shape—the shape the crystalline lens assumes with both eyes open.
- The visual acuity test can reveal which eye is weaker even if the patient's prescription for each eye is the same or almost the same. The information determines the wearing sequence in Step 7. It is important to know which contact lens to wear first or which eye performs the drill first.

14.4   STEP 3

14.4.1   MEASURE THE CORNEA CURVATURE

If you have a keratometer, measure the horizontal and vertical curvature of the cornea. The k readings are expressed in diopters. (Refer to the *Addendum* for more information on taking a k reading.) If you do not have a keratometer, the patient can request a k reading from an eye care specialist. The measurement does not necessarily have to be taken by a private optometrist. It can also be taken by an optician or an optometrist at a retail optical outlet such as Costco or Walmart.

14.5   STEP 4

14.5.1   DETERMINE THE MID K

Calculate the mid k (which is the average of the horizontal and vertical curvatures) by adding the measurements for the horizontal and vertical curvatures and dividing the sum by two. The mid k represents the average curvature of the cornea. It is over a small area. When the curve is extended, it represents the area covered by the contact lens. The lens that you would order is flatter than mid k to enable a "contact lens draw."

14.6   STEP 5

14.6.1   CALCULATE THE BASE CURVE

14.6.1.1   THE FLATNESS FACTOR

The lens' flatness represents its base curve. The base curve refers to the inside curvature of the contact lens. It is designed slightly flatter or less curved than the mid k you calculated in Step 4—but it is not as flat as an ortho K lens. It represents the curve required to establish emmetropia.

The flatness factor is generally equal to the absolute value (without regard to the plus or minus sign) of the prescription. If the prescription is −0.50 D, for example, the flatness factor is 0.50 D. The flatness factor is subtracted from the dioptric mid k calculated in Step 4 to determine the base curve. If the mid k is 43.25 D, for example, the base curve of the ortho C lens would be 43.25 D minus 0.50 D or 42.75 D. You would subtract 0.50 D from the mid k instead of adding it because you want to make the lens flatter. Remember, in reference to measurements in diopters, a flatter lens is represented by a decrease in value, whereas in reference to measurements in millimeters of radius, a flatter lens is represented by an increase in value. (The flatness factor as outlined in the *Specifications* indicates how flat the lens should be from the mid k for a specific prescription.)

From the conversion table, this base curve can also be expressed as 7.90 mm. When you are ordering from a lab or from a supplier online, always give them the measurements in millimeters of radius. (Refer to the *Specifications* for the diopters to millimeters of radius conversion table.)

14.6.1.2   MILD MYOPIA WITH THE SAME PRESCRIPTION IN BOTH EYES

If the patient has mild myopia from −0.50 D to −0.75 D and the prescription is the same for both eyes, the lens' flatness is equivalent to the absolute value of the patient's prescription for the sphere of the right and left eye. (Refer to the flatness factor chart in the *Specifications* and to the chapter *Treating Mild and Moderate Myopia* for the definition of the "sphere.") The base curve of a lens for a client with a prescription of −0.75 D for each eye and with a mid k as in the example above would be 43.25 D minus 0.75 D or 42.50 D. From the diopters to millimeters of radius conversion table in the *Specifications*, the base curve can also be expressed as 7.94 mm. (The mid k for each eye is usually different, but for the purpose of illustration suppose it is the same.)

14.6.1.3   MODERATE MYOPIA WITH THE SAME PRESCRIPTION IN BOTH EYES

If the patient has moderate myopia from −1.00 D to −1.75 D and the prescription is the same for both eyes, the lens' flatness is equivalent to the absolute value of the patient's prescription for the sphere of the right and left eye. The base curve of a lens for a client with a prescription of −1.50 D for each eye and with a mid k as in the example above would be 43.25 D minus 1.50 D or 41.75 D. From the conversion table, the base curve can also be expressed as 8.08 mm. If you compare this lens to the lens of the patient with mild myopia, you would find that the lens for the moderate myopic eye is flatter. A 8.08-mm lens is flatter than a 7.94-mm lens—the lens fitted for a mild myopic client in the previous example. With measurements expressed in millimeters, the higher the number, the flatter the lens.

The crystalline lens and sclera of a moderate myopic eye deviated more compared to a mild myopic eye and needs a flatter lens to address it. A flatter lens would "loosen" the oblique muscles more to stimulate the ciliary muscle to relax more. It requires a higher "contact lens draw" to alter the curvature of the sclera as well as the lens.

14.6.1.4   A DISPARITY OF −0.25 D

If the difference in the prescription between the right and left eye is −0.25 D, the flatness factor is still equivalent to the absolute value of the prescription for the right and left eye. The disparity in prescription is within the margin of error that allows the flatness factor to be equal to the absolute value of the patient's prescription. For example, if the patient's prescription is OD −0.50 D and OS −0.75 D, the lens' flatness for the right eye is 0.50 D and for the left eye is 0.75 D. (Refer to the *Specifications*.)

14.6.1.5   A DISPARITY OF −0.50 D

If the difference in the prescriptions between the right and left eye is −0.50 D, the disparity is outside the margin of error that allows the flatness factor to be equal to the patient's prescription. The flatness factor for the better eye is 0.25 D more than the absolute value of the prescription for that eye. The lens' flatness for the weaker eye is 0.25 D less than the absolute value of the prescription for that eye. For example, if the prescription is OD −1.00 D and OS −1.50 D, the flatness for the right eye is 1.25 D and for the left eye is 1.25 D. (Refer to the *Specifications*.)

14.6.1.6   A DISPARITY OF −0.75 D

A disparity of −0.75 D may still qualify as anisometropia—especially if one eye is in the mild range and the other eye is in the moderate range. In those ranges, the patient is more sensitive to the discrepancy than someone with severe myopia. The flatness factor of the lenses for both eyes is equivalent to the absolute value of the prescription of the weaker eye. For example, if the patient's prescription is OD −1.00 D and OS −1.75 D, the flatness factor for the right and left eye is 1.75 D. The maximum flatness would be 2.0 D if the weaker eye is in the midrange. If the patient's prescription is OD −1.50 D and OS −2.25 D, for example, the flatness factor for the right and left eye is 2.00 D regardless of the prescription of the weaker eye (with midrange myopia from −2.00 D to −2.75 D). Do not go beyond −2.00 D.

14.6.1.7   A DISPARITY OF −1.00 D (ANISOMETROPIA)

Anisometropia refers to the difference in the prescription between the right and left eye of −1.00 D or more. If the prescription of one eye is mild or moderate and the other eye is in the moderate range, the flatness factor for both lenses takes on the absolute value of the prescription of the weaker eye. For example, if the right eye is −0.50 D and the other eye is −1.50 D, then the flatness factor for the right and left lens is 1.50 D. If one eye's prescription is moderate and the other eye is in the midrange, the flatness factor for both lenses is 2.00 D. For example, if the right eye is −1.00

D and the other eye is −2.25 D, then the flatness factor for the right and left lens is 2.00 D regardless of the prescription of the weaker eye (with midrange myopia from −2.00 D to −2.75 D).

14.6.1.8   A PRESCRIPTION OF −0.25 D FOR BOTH EYES

I suggest you pass up on treating a patient with a prescription of −0.25 D in both eyes (or in one eye). It is more difficult to treat than the higher ranges of myopia. The deviation is closer to the emmetropic state than other ranges of myopia. There is not much room for error. It is easy to overcorrect the crystalline lens' or the eye's deviation by exceeding the required flatness. You can only reinstate the neuromuscular message of the normal eye—not beyond normal. (Refer to the chapters *Troubleshooting* and *Treating Mild and Moderate Myopia* for more information.)

The patient can attempt natural relaxation drills instead. Most of the deviation is in the crystalline lens, and those drills target the ciliary muscle directly. (Refer to the *Addendum.*) Also inform the patient to avoid any bad habits which can trigger and increase in "effort to see." (Refer to the chapters *Extraneous Variables, Mental Strain,* and *The Effort to See.*)

14.6.1.9   ASTIGMATISM

If the patient has astigmatism plus mild or moderate myopia and if the astigmatism is −1.00 D or less, do not adjust the lens' flatness to treat mild or moderate myopia. The flatness factor is equivalent to the patient's prescription. If the patient has astigmatism plus mild or moderate myopia and if the astigmatism is more than −1.00 D, make an adjustment flatter than the required flatness factor. Refer to the *Specifications* for the amount of adjustment according to the severity of the astigmatism.

14.6.1.10   PRESBYOPIA

If the patient has presbyopia and mild or moderate myopia, the presbyopia should be less than the absolute value of the "sphere." If it is less than the absolute value of the "sphere," then the lens' flatness is equal to the patient's prescription. If it is equal to or more than the absolute value to the "sphere," you would have to treat the refractive error as presbyopia.

The treatment is beyond the scope of this book and would be covered in a different publication.

14.6.1.11   REPLACING AN ORTHO C LENS

If the patient lost the ortho C lenses, another practitioner, even someone experienced in ortho C, would have difficulty replacing the lenses. The lens was determined by the original prescription before the treatment. If the patient had severe myopia, for example, and if she reduced her nearsightedness by ortho C, she cannot go by her reduced prescription to order a new lens. The base curve would be different. The improvement in visual acuity means that the lens is less flat compared to the original lens. You have to go by the original prescription even when the eye became emmetropic. The base curve of that lens is the curve the myopic eye strives to attain. Once the eye achieves that curvature, the patient wears the lens regularly to maintain emmetropia. A different base curve will make the visual acuity worse.

You should give the client the specifications in case you would not be available to order a replacement lens. When ordering online, there is no slot to allow the patient to specify the lens' thickness. The thickness must be 0.15 mm thick. The "comments" section, or equivalent, is probably the only spot to request that specification. Ordering from an eye care specialist ensures that the thickness is correct.

14.7   STEP 6

14.7.1   DETERMINE THE WEAKER EYE

You need to know which eye is the weaker eye to determine the wearing sequence. The wearing sequence in any drill is important (which eye wears the lens first when wearing the lenses one at a time or which eye performs the drill first with both lenses on). Wearing the lens or performing the drill in the correct sequence maximizes the patient's improvement in visual acuity. You would perform the wearing sequence test in the next step. A hint in determining the weaker eye is the patient's prescription or the visual acuity measurements.

14.7.1.1 FROM THE DIFFERENCE IN PRESCRIPTION

If there is a difference in prescription between each eye, the "weaker eye" is the eye with the higher prescription. If the prescription of the right eye is −0.75 D and the left eye is −1.25 D, the weaker eye is most likely the left eye.

14.7.1.2 FROM THE VISUAL ACUITY MEASUREMENT

If the prescription of each eye is different, then the visual acuity test in Step 2 would confirm the weaker eye. If the prescription of each eye is the same, a visual acuity test can still determine the weaker eye when the crystalline lens participates in focusing. During a conventional eye exam, it was probably bypassed. The weaker eye is the eye that reads the least number of lines on the Snellen chart. If the prescription for both eyes is −1.25 D, and the right eye is capable of reading up to line 5 on the Snellen chart while the left eye can only read up to line 4, the weaker eye is the left eye. If the visual acuity test with the naked eye cannot determine the weaker eye, then place a −0.50 D trial lens in front of each eye. It should relax the ciliary muscle sufficiently to allow the better eye to respond better than the weaker eye.

14.7.2 BREAK

Order the ortho C lenses. If you have not done so, order the glasses for your inventory. Have the client come back in about a week or two. Tell anyone who wears glasses all the time to rely less on them during this period. It is easier for the mild and moderate myopee to alter the habit compared to someone with a higher range of nearsightedness. Tell the patient to resort to the glasses only under adverse conditions: driving, taking notes from the blackboard, making out what is projected in a dark room, etc. Do not wear them to read, to work on the computer, or to watch TV. It is okay to wear them for driving a vehicle because objects in the distance are over 20 ft away. The rays of light from an object of regard are parallel. Thus the focal point falls on the retina instead of behind the retina (when looking at objects closer than 20 ft).

Inform your client the benefits of natural relaxation exercises prior to prolong work in front of a computer or when there is a feeling that fatigue is about to set in. But do not perform them immediately before or after performing the drills with the ortho C lenses. It neurologically interferes with the outcome. (For a description on palming and swinging, refer to the *Addendum*.)

14.8   STEP 7

14.8.1   DETERMINE THE WEARING SEQUENCE

14.8.1.1   THE WEARING SEQUENCE TEST

Each drill requires a specific wearing sequence in terms of which lens to wear first. Once you know which eye is the better eye and which eye is weaker, the correct wearing sequence becomes predictable. However, you still have to confirm it. The Wearing Sequence Test is a low-intensity test, and it is suitable for any type of refractive error. It does not interfere with the actual drill the client should be doing. If the patient's vision becomes blurred after the test, it is an indication that the wearing sequence is incorrect. The blurriness is not permanent. The decline in visual acuity would reverse once you determine the correct sequence. The patient would wear the lenses in the proper sequence starting with the weaker eye first.

Perform the Wearing Sequence Test as follows:

1.   Insert the lens for the weaker eye first (the eye determined to be weaker in Step 6),
2.   Perform the Distance Drill. (Refer to the chapter *What to Do* for information on the supplementary drills.)
3.   Then remove the lens and take a binocular and monocular visual acuity test with the naked eye (and with the weaker glasses if applicable).
4.   Insert the other lens for the better eye.
5.   Perform the Distance Drill.
6.   Then remove the lens and take a binocular and monocular visual acuity test with the naked eye (and with the weaker glasses if applicable).

Perform the visual acuity test quickly in Step 3 so that the client retains the relaxation from the drill prior to performing Step 4. Although only one lens was on (on the weaker eye), it also stimulates the other eye that did not have the lens on (the better eye). There will be an improvement in visual acuity in each eye (Yee, 2011).

The patient's visual acuity should further improve after performing the Distance Drill with the lens on the better eye. For example, after the patient did the drill with the lens on the weaker eye, there may be a one-line improvement binocularly; and after doing the drill again with the lens in the better eye, there should be an improvement of another line binocularly. Your binocular vision is the determining factor—not your monocular vision. A binocular improvement of two lines or more after the first application means that the eye is receptive to ortho C and that most of the refractive error resides in the lens. Do not reverse the sequence. Otherwise the patient would see worse.

Sometimes there may be little difference in visual acuity after the test. You can still assume that the wearing sequence is correct. A lower than expected improvement means that there is a partial resistance to ortho C— either because the eyeball deviated slightly more or a partial spasticity has set in to restrict the lens from becoming flatter. I had participants who did not respond to the test but had excellent results after the Second Resistance Test. The steps of the Wearing Sequence Test are also similar to the First Resistance Test. You are actually performing both tests at the same time. (Refer to the resistance tests in the next step for more information.)

14.8.1.2 REVERSE THE WEARING SEQUENCE

There is the possibility that the weaker eye may be more receptive to ortho C than the better eye. It rarely happens, but there are instances where the higher myopic eye is more receptive to ortho C. You would then have the patient reverse the standard sequence by wearing the lens in the better eye first and finishing with the lens in the weaker eye instead.

The following scenario is a hint that the regular wearing sequence should be reversed: Suppose the prescription is the same for each eye. After wearing the lens in what you thought was the weaker eye and performing the Distance Drill, the client experienced a two line increase on the Snellen chart; but there was a one line decrease after wearing the lens and performing the drill in the better eye. Do not be concerned with the regression. The test allows for a negative outcome. Unlike other extraneous variables, it is not permanent. (Refer to the chapter *Extraneous Variables* for more information.)

To reverse the relapse, the patient does not have to start all over again. He or she just needs to insert the other lens back on the other eye. For example, if the result of wearing the right lens first and then the left was problematic after performing the Distance Drill, then just wear the right lens again and perform the Distance Drill. If the visual acuity improves, then you know that the proper sequence is wearing the left lens first and then right.

But if reversing the wearing sequence makes the visual acuity worse again, you would have to revert back to the previous sequence to reset the client's visual acuity to the way it was prior to any drill—by wearing the left lens again. A decrease in visual acuity twice in a row is an indication that the lenses (or lens) are too flat. You either overcorrected something or corrected something that does not need any correction. When wearing the left lens again, it resets or partially reset the decline in visual acuity. Check the calculation for the lens' flatness factor.

For the last 30 years or so, the Wearing Sequence Test I performed was always straightforward. The only problem I had was when the prescription for each eye is −0.25 D. It is easy to exceed the required flatness factor. (Refer to the chapter *Troubleshooting* for an example of such a problem.) Also be aware that some first time wearers of RGP lenses may not show a proper response to ortho C until the second or third application. The eye naturally rejects any foreign object in the eye, and there can be a lot of tearing. The eye would adapt to the lens by the second or third application.

14.8.1.3   REVERSE THE WEARING SEQUENCE FOR COMPOUND ANISOMETROPIA AND ANISOMETROPIC AMBLYOPIA

The other exception to the rule is when the patient has compound aniso-metropia and anisometropic amblyopia. You reverse the normal sequence by wearing the lens in the better eye first and finishing with the lens in the weaker eye instead. It is not because the weaker eye is more receptive to ortho C than the better eye. The neuropathway is different. (Refer to the chapter *Treating Anisometropia* for more information.)

14.9   STEP 8

14.9.1   PERFORM THE RESISTANCE TESTS

14.9.1.1   TESTING AN EYE WITH A PRIMARY REFRACTIVE ERROR

If a patient has a primary refractive error, perform the resistance tests to determine if the eye has a partial resistance. If there is a partial resistance, the eye is slightly outside the myopic model. The Standard Drill would not work. You have to resort to another drill.

14.9.1.2   A LOW RESISTANCE

Perform The First and Second Resistance Test as described in the chapter *The Theory Behind the Resistance Tests*. You can expect an eye with a primary refractive error with a low resistance to improve by approximately two lines on the Snellen chart after the First Resistance Test and another one line after the Second Resistance Test. If the response is as expected, the patient would perform the recommended drill as listed in Step 9.

14.9.1.3   A PARTIAL RESISTANCE

If an eye has a partial resistance but outside the myopic model, one possible outcome is that there is about a one line gain after the First Resistance Test and possibly about another line after the Second Resistance Test. Another possible outcome is that there is no response to the First Resistance Test, but it may respond dramatically to the Second Resistance Test. A final possible outcome is that there is no response to the First, Second, or Third Resistance Test, but it may respond marginally to the Fourth Resistance Test. Once you identified the partial resistance, refer the patient to Step 10 for the recommended drill for the specific problem. The drill is different from the recommended drill in Step 9. Those drills are for an eye with a low resistance or partial resistance within the myopic model.

14.9.1.4   A HIGH RESISTANCE

If there is no sign of any improvement in visual acuity after you conducted all the tests, ask the client if he wants to continue. Most likely spasticity has set in. To relax the ciliary muscle, he would have to depend less on the glasses and perform certain relaxation exercises such as palming, swinging, and stretching to eliminate the spasm and to gain some depth perception before attempting the treatment again. (Refer to *Treating the Loss of Depth Perception* and to the *Addendum* for more information.)

14.9.1.5   *TESTING AN EYE WITH A SECONDARY REFRACTIVE ERROR*

If the patient has a secondary refractive error, you are performing the resistance tests not to determine if the eye has a partial resistance. You already know that there is a partial resistance. There is another refractive error on top of the myopia. It is treatable because it is within the myopic model. Instead you are relying on the tests to give you more information on borderline cases and to determine which drill is more effective.

If you are addressing secondary refractive errors within the myopic model, a resistance test can assist you with treating compound astigmatism which borders on the possibility of high astigmatism. The First Resistance Test can determine which drill is appropriate, the Standard Drill or Modified Preliminary Drill, in borderline myopia and astigmatism.

14.9.1.6   *BORDERLINE MYOPIA AND ASTIGMATISM*

The First Resistance Test provides valuable information for the patient with borderline myopia and astigmatism. When the sphere is moderate and the astigmatism is 50% of the sphere such as $-1.00-0.50 \times 180$, the outcome of the First Resistance Test can offer a hint as to which drill is more effective: the Standard Drill or Modified Preliminary Drill. You need to know whether to treat the myopia by applying the Standard Drill or the astigmatism by applying the Modified Preliminary Drill. If the eye does not respond to the First Resistance Test, try the Modified Preliminary Drill. It should be noted that the Wearing Sequence Test is similar to the First Resistance Test. A compound astigmatic eye may not respond to the Wearing Sequence Test. You would have to go by the prescription or the visual acuity test if the prescriptions for both eyes are the same.

14.10   STEP 9

14.10.1   THE RECOMMENDED DRILLS FOR A LOW OR PARTIAL RESISTANCE EYE WITHIN THE MYOPIC MODEL

The following are the recommended drills for an eye within the myopic model with a low resistance or partial resistance:

- *Mild myopia of −0.50 D with the same prescription in both eyes*
  The treatment: The Modified Preliminary Drill.

- *Mild and moderate myopia from −0.75 D to −1.75 D with the same prescription in both the eyes*
  The treatment: The Standard Drill.

- *Mild and moderate myopia from −0.75D to −1.75 D with a disparity of −0.25 D*
  The treatment: The Standard Drill.

- *Mild and moderate myopia from −0.75 D to −1.75 D with a disparity of −0.50 D*
  The treatment: The Modified Preliminary Drill.

- *Mild and moderate myopia from −0.75 D to −1.75 D with a disparity of −0.75 D*
  The treatment: Perform the Preliminary Drill first and then the Modified Preliminary Drill.

- *Mild, moderate, and midrange myopia with a disparity of −1.00 D or more*
  The treatment: Perform the Preliminary Drill first and then the Modified Preliminary Drill.

- *Mild or moderate myopia with low astigmatism*
  The treatment: The Standard Drill.

- *Mild or moderate myopia with high astigmatism*
  The treatment: The Modified Preliminary Drill.

- *Simple astigmatism*
  The treatment: The Modified Preliminary Drill.

- *Anisometropia with high astigmatism*
  The treatment: The Modified Preliminary Drill.

- *Anisometropia with Anisometropic Amblyopia*
  The treatment: The Modified Preliminary Drill

14.11   STEP 10

14.11.1   THE RECOMMENDED DRILLS FOR A PARTIAL RESISTANCE EYE OUTSIDE THE MYOPIC MODEL

The following are the recommended drills for an eye outside the myopic model with a partial resistance given its response to the different resistance tests:

14.11.1.1   FIRST SCENARIO (PARTIAL RESPONSE AFTER THE FIRST AND SECOND RESISTANCE TEST)

There is about a one-line improvement after the First Resistance Test and about another one line after the Second Resistance Test. The following is the recommended drill given the myopic range and disparity:

Mild and moderate myopia from −0.75 D to −1.75 D with the same prescription in both the eyes or with a disparity of −0.25 D.

The treatment: Perform the Modified Standard Drill first for 2 weeks (two to three times a week). Then perform the Modified Preliminary Drill.

Refer to the *Addendum* on how to perform the relaxation, swinging, and stretching drills. You may have to fit the patient with a pair of weaker glasses in the interim. Test with the trial lenses or glasses from your inventory. The power is undercorrected by two lines on the Snellen chart if you expect the visual acuity of the patient to improve by two lines in the short to medium term. (Refer to the sections on Visual Acuity Test and Providing a Visual Aid in the Interim in the *Addendum*.)

Provide the patient with a list of possible factors that may contribute to a partial spasm. (Refer to the chapter *The Effort to See*.) Inform the patient about the different exercises and behavior changes (such as adjusting the distance for the reading range and midrange) to deal with the loss in depth perception. (Refer to the chapter *Treating a Loss of Depth Perception* for more information.) When the patient is ready, determine the retention period. (Refer to the chapter *Wearing Schedule*.)

14.11.1.2   SECOND SCENARIO (RESPONSIVE JUST TO THE SECOND RESISTANCE TEST)

The patient does not respond to the First Resistance Test, but there is an improvement of two to three lines after the Second Resistance Test. The following is the recommended drill given the myopic range and disparity:

Mild and moderate myopia from −0.75 D to −1.75 D with the same prescription in both the eyes or with a disparity of −0.25 D.

The treatment: Perform the Preliminary Drill first for 2 weeks (two to three times a week). Then perform the Modified Preliminary Drill. Also try the Standard Drill the next day. From the before and after results, determine which drill is more suitable.

Refer to the *Addendum* on how to perform the relaxation, swinging, and stretching drills. You may have to fit the patient with a pair of weaker glasses in the interim. Test with the trial lenses or glasses from your inventory. The power is undercorrected by two lines on the Snellen chart if you expect the visual acuity of the patient to improve by two lines in the short to medium term. (Refer to the sections on Visual Acuity Test and Providing a Visual Aid in the Interim in the *Addendum*.)

Provide the patient with a list of possible factors that may contribute to a partial spasm. (Refer to the chapter *The Effort to See*.) Inform the patient about the different exercises and behavior changes (such as adjusting the distance for the reading range and midrange) to deal with the loss in depth perception. (Refer to the chapter *Treating a Loss of Depth Perception* for more information.) When the patient is ready, determine the retention period. (Refer to the chapter *Wearing Schedule*.)

14.11.1.3   THIRD SCENARIO (RESPONSIVE JUST TO THE FOURTH RESISTANCE TEST)

The patient does not respond to the First, Second, or Third Resistance Test. There is about a one-line improvement after the Fourth Resistance Test and about another one line after performing the recommended drill. The following is the recommended drill given the specific refractive errors and disparities:

Mild and moderate myopia from −0.75 D to −1.75 D with the same prescription in both the eyes or with a disparity of −0.25 D

The treatment: Perform the Modified Standard Drill first for 2 weeks (two to three times a week). Then perform the Modified Preliminary Drill.

Refer to the *Addendum* on how to perform the relaxation, swinging, and stretching drills. You may have to fit the patient with a pair of weaker glasses in the interim. Test with the trial lenses or glasses from your inventory. The power is undercorrected by two lines on the Snellen chart if you expect the visual acuity of the patient to improve by two lines in the short to medium term. (Refer to the sections on Visual Acuity Test and Providing a Visual Aid in the Interim in the *Addendum*.)

Provide the patient with a list of possible factors that may contribute to a partial spasm. (Refer to the chapter *The Effort to See*.) Inform the patient about the different exercises and behavior changes (such as adjusting the distance for the reading range and midrange) to deal with the loss in depth perception. (Refer to the chapter *Treating a Loss of Depth Perception* for more information.) When the patient is ready, determine the retention period. (Refer to the chapter *Wearing Schedule*.)

14.12   STEP 11

14.12.1   SCHEDULE A FOLLOW-UP

For a low resistance eye or partial resistance eye within the myopic model, have the client perform the drill two times a week for 1 week. For a partial resistance eye outside the myopic mode, have the client perform the drill two to three times a week for 2 weeks. Schedule a follow-up afterwards to check the client's retention in visual acuity. You would also check for other things as well—as listed in the chapter *Follow-Ups*. If everything checks out, have the client perform the drill one more time at the clinic. Ask the client to help you determine the retention period by keeping track of how long the improvement lasts. (Refer to the chapter *Wearing Schedule* for more information.)

KEYWORDS

- pupil distance
- Snellen chart
- keratometer reading
- mid k
- extraneous variable
- visual acuity test
- diopter

CHAPTER 15

THE THEORY BEHIND THE RESISTANCE TESTS (IT'S NOT JUST A TEST)

ABSTRACT

The treatment is optimal if the myopia is within the myopic model. It is still possible, however, to treat myopia slightly outside of it. There are some participants, for example, who tried their best to keep the ciliary muscle pliable except for the few times when they did something out of the ordinary—such as wearing contact lenses to play sports. Although it may have occurred less than a dozen times a year, it was enough to create a partial resistance. The directly induced stress induced a partial spasm.

You can refer to the resistance tests as a flow chart to help you identify the type of resistance encountered by the myopic eye. You start by testing a patient with the First Resistance Test. If you suspect a partial resistance, you would continue with the other tests only if he has a primary refractive error—not a secondary refractive error. A primary refractive error refers to mild and moderate myopia with the same prescription in each eye or with a disparity less than −0.50 D. The other types of refractive errors are considered secondary refractive errors, such as: anisometropia, compound anisometropia and anisometropic amblyopia, and compound myopia and astigmatism where the astigmatism is high. The Third and Fourth Resistance Tests are not compatible with the actual drill assigned to a secondary refractive error since the Third and Fourth Resistance Tests together make up the Standard Drill. The Standard Drill is more applicable to refractive errors that allow for the multiplier effect in the first part of the drill. Secondary refractive errors generally prefer a less intense stimulation by wearing one lens at a time to induce an indirect effect.

However, there is an exception. If you are addressing secondary refractive errors within the myopic model, the First Resistance Test can determine whether to apply the Standard Drill or Modified Preliminary Drill when treating borderline myopia and high astigmatism. You are not checking for a partial resistance. You already know there is a partial resistance due to the presence of astigmatism as well as myopia. Instead, you are actually testing the astigmatism's intensity level. If it is high, it would not respond to the First Resistance Test.

15.1   IT'S NOT JUST A TEST

The resistance tests are not just tests per se but are also possibilities for unlocking the partial spasm incurred by the ciliary muscle. Once it is unlocked, it provides a hint of the eye's resistance level by assessing how much improvement was gained and which test induced just the right stimulation. Once you removed the partial resistance, refer the patient to Step 10 in *The Procedure* for the recommended drill for the specific problem. The drill is different from the recommended drill in Step 9. Those drills were designed for an eye with a low resistance or an eye with a partial resistance but still within the myopic model.

15.2   THE RESISTANCE OF THE EYE

If a primary refractive error falls within the myopic model, it has a low resistance. The assumption is that the crystalline lens would deviate more than the eyeball. An eye with a low resistance suggests that myopia mainly resides in the crystalline lens. If it responds favorably to the First and Second Resistance Test, you would then proceed to the actual drill: the Standard Drill. The Standard Drill attends to a standard deviation (where the lens' deviation is due to an indirect restriction imposed by the oblique muscles), and that is why I call it the Standard Drill.

If the eye has a partial resistance, it can still be within the myopic model or it can fall slightly outside of it. If it falls within the myopic model, it is probably due to another refractive error on top of mild or moderate myopia. A secondary refractive error such as anisometropia is still correctable. However, some types of myopia and astigmatism are borderline secondary refractive errors. You can test the resistance of the astigmatism to determine which drill is more effective.

If the partial resistance falls outside the myopic model, it can either display features of a primary refractive error or secondary refractive error. It suggests that the ciliary muscle incurred a partial spasm due to a direct influence—from a pair of glasses or contact lenses. for example, and as a result, the eyeball may deviate more than the crystalline lens. You would not know if the ciliary muscle is partially seized until you conduct the resistance tests. If the eye has a high resistance, ciliary muscle spasm had set in. (Refer to the chapter *Treating the Loss of Depth Perception* for more information on the direct and indirect influence of near-point stress.)

15.2.1   THE THEORY ON TREATING AN EYE WITH A LOW RESISTANCE AND WITH A PARTIAL RESISTANCE

15.2.1.1   A LOW RESISTANCE

Besides ranking the eye's resistance, each resistance test sets up different conditions to activate the ciliary muscle. If the eye has a primary refractive error, a low resistance, and within the myopic model, the ciliary muscle can be activated to relax under the right conditions to flatten out the lens—or more specifically, the occluded neutral shape of the lens. In turn, it would stimulate the rectus muscles to tighten up to alter the myopic shape of the eyeball. The eyeball can only flatten for distant focusing when the lens flattens.

The phenomenon is the opposite of near-point stress where the eyeball becomes elongated when the lens makes an excessive effort to perform work at the near range. By introducing certain conditions where the crystalline lens needs to maintain the focus of something far away, it may entice the eyeball to become less elongated to alleviate the effort. The ciliary muscle does not make an excessive effort; otherwise, it would trigger an "excessive effort to see." It is just the right amount. It depends on the resistance of the ciliary muscle. It is the excessive tension of the oblique muscles that restricts how much the ciliary muscle can relax. If I create a condition where I can relax the oblique muscles sufficiently to stimulate the ciliary muscle, it may also stimulate the rectus muscles to tighten to reduce the elongated eye due to the common neural pathway.

15.2.1.2   A PARTIAL RESISTANCE

If the eye has a primary refractive error and a partial resistance which displaces it slightly outside the myopic model, it is possible to relax the ciliary muscle in the same manner to activate the eyeball to become less elongated. The setting that is right for the low resistance eye is not appropriate for the partial resistance eye. You have to find another condition for the patient to allow a "contact lens draw" to produce a partial reversal. You have to find which resistance test produces the right condition.

As you conduct each test, you are changing the intensity of each resistance test incrementally. When it is low, it implies flattening the crystalline lens less in order to entice the eyeball to flatten. When it is high, it attempts to flatten the crystalline lens differently in order to entice the eyeball to flatten. You are not increasing or decreasing the pressure or a force of any kind. You want to find the right setting to enable the lens to flatten and the eyeball to retract. When the eye is slightly outside the myopic model, the eyeball may have deviated more than the lens; and partial spasticity of the ciliary muscle may have set in. You have to influence the lens in the right amount before the eyeball can respond.

Unlike a low resistance eye, a partial resistance eye would respond only to certain resistance tests. If the eyeball deviated partially compared to the lens, there would be a partial response to the First and Second Resistance Test. In some cases, it would respond to the Second Resistance Test even though there is no response to the First Resistance Test. If the eyeball deviated more, the Fourth Resistance Test would deal with it even though there is no response to the other resistance tests.

An eye with a partial resistance needs to be treated in a special way by resorting to another drill. The patient would also need to continue relaxing the ciliary muscle by other means. Ortho C does not attend to the partial spasticity causing the partial resistance. If there is a total resistance, however, the patient would have to alleviate the spasm before attempting ortho C. (Refer to the chapter *Treating the Loss of Depth Perception* for more information.)

15.2.2   MINI DRILLS

The tests are actually mini drills to jump-start the ciliary muscle. The crystalline lens needs to change first before the sclera can change. Each test is like a defibrillator set at different intensities to activate the ciliary muscle. Although the test can be regarded as a drill, it does not replace the recommended drill assigned to the specific problem. If the eye responds to a specific test, a resistance can build up if the patient continues to rely on it instead of the actual drill.

15.2.3   DEMONSTRATING THE THEORY

If the myopic eye is −1.00 D, for example, that amount of tension is attributed to the oblique muscles. It locks in the myopic shape of the lens and the eyeball. To unlock it, you need to loosen the oblique muscles by 1.00 D. If a partial resistance sets in, the direct stress initially tightens the ciliary muscle. The refractive error may still be −1.00, but the tension of the ciliary muscle that locks in the myopic shape of the lens is higher. Later, the oblique muscles pick up the excessive tension, and it may also be reflected in the elongated eyeball.

The patient may not be aware of the deterioration since she still sees close to 20/20 with the −1.00 D glasses. If her visual acuity without glasses is (OU) line 3, it is a hint that the eyeball also deviated more than usual. A low resistance eye would see around line 5 when tested in a room with adequate light to allow the lens to participate. Without the assistance of the crystalline lens (i.e., in a dim room with the chart projected), she should see down to line 4 prior to the increase in tension of the oblique muscles. (Refer to the *Addendum* for the Snellen chart reading to diopter conversion.) If her visual acuity deteriorated to line 3 when tested in a room with adequate light, it means the crystalline lens did not participate in the test due to the tension of the ciliary muscle; and the eyeball had elongated. You would probably get the same results after testing her in a dim lit room.

15.3   TESTING THE RESISTANCE OF A PRIMARY REFRACTIVE ERROR

There are four resistance tests to determine the resistance level of an eye with a primary refractive error. The First Resistance Test is equivalent to the first part of the Preliminary Drill, and the Second Resistance Test is equivalent to the second part of the Preliminary Drill. The Third

Resistance Test is equivalent to the first part of the Standard Drill, and Fourth Resistance Test is equivalent to the second part of the Standard Drill. Each successive test is an increase in intensity.

The outcome of a specific test is an indication of the ciliary muscle's ability to bring a distant object into focus; and that in turn indicates the ciliary muscle's flexibility. Its flexibility represents the resistance of the eye as a whole since the eyeball cannot shift until the lens shift. You would have the patient conducting each test until it activates a response.

15.3.1   FIRST RESISTANCE TEST

Once your client finish the First Resistance Test, instruct him to continue with the Second Resistance Test afterwards. It is as if he was performing the Preliminary Drill. A patient with −1.25 D in both eyes, for example, can perform those tests even though the Standard Drill is the drill of choice. Although the prescription is the same for both eyes, a visual acuity test would reveal the weaker eye. If the eye responds favorably to the First Resistance Test according to the proper wearing sequence, it should also respond favorably to the Second Resistance Test; and if the eye responds favorably to the Preliminary Drill, it should respond favorably to the Standard Drill.

15.3.1.1   A TYPICAL RESPONSE FROM A LOW RESISTANCE EYE

Perform the First Resistance Test as outlined at the end of the chapter. When a low resistance eye responds well to the low intensity test, it entices the crystalline lens to flatten out as much as possible. The "focal point draw" stimulates the lens' open neutral shape. It is already a bit flat. If the lens is flexible (due to the flexibility of the ciliary muscle), the drill would flatten the lens further to the extent that it can compensate not only its own myopic shape but also the eyeball's myopic shape. It is an indication that most of the myopia resides in the lens. Only an eye restricted indirectly by near-point stress can allow such a "shift." You can expect a two-line improvement on average after performing the First Resistance Test and another one line after the Second Resistance Test.

Refer to the chapter *The Procedure* under the section *The Recommended Drills for a Low Resistance Eye* for the drill that the patient should be doing given the specific refractive error. In this case, it would be the Standard Drill. Perform that drill for two or three times a week for 2 weeks. Then refer to the *Wearing Schedule* to determine the retention period.

15.3.1.2 FIRST POSSIBLE RESPONSE FROM A PARTIAL RESISTANCE EYE

If there is a partial response of one line or less on the Snellen chart after the First Resistance Test, complete the Second Resistance Test. The patient must perform the Second Resistance Test afterwards to maximize the possible outcome. The First and Second Resistance Test makes up the Preliminary Drill. The myopic eye with a partial resistance may gain less than one line after the Second Resistance Test.

15.3.2 SECOND RESISTANCE TEST

Different conditions are set up in the Second Resistance Test. To ensure the lens flattens partially, the Snellen chart is hung in artificial light. It is more challenging than conducting the drill in natural light. During the test, one eye is occluded. Monocular vision is more challenging than binocular vision for the myopic eye. If the conditions were not that challenging, the lens alone will bring everything into focus as in the First Resistance Test since the object of regard is just 5 ft away.

The outcome of the Second Resistance Test is contingent on performing the First Resistance Test. If the patient took too long checking the visual acuity after the First Resistance Test, it may interfere with the outcome of the Second Resistance Test. In that case, start the First Resistance Test all over again from Step 1. The patient is actually performing the Preliminary Drill from Steps 1 to 4.

Even if there was no response after conducting the First Resistance Test, it is still required before proceeding to the next test. The first test prepares the eye for the second test by "loosening" the oblique muscles. Perhaps relaxing the spasm of the ciliary muscle needs to occur in stages. You cannot have the patient just perform the Second Resistance Test by itself if you suspect a partial resistance. It would not work.

15.3.2.1   FIRST POSSIBLE RESPONSE FROM A PARTIAL RESISTANCE EYE (CONTINUING FROM THE FIRST RESISTANCE TEST)

If the patient experiences a partial improvement of about one line or less after the First Resistance Test, there may also be an improvement of one line or less after the Second Resistance Test. It suggests that the partial spasm of the ciliary muscle only allowed a partial reversal of the lens and eyeball. Although the crystalline lens deviated in the proper proportion compared to the eyeball, the partial spasticity reduced how much the lens can flatten. Since it responded to the First and Second Resistance Test, the degree of spasticity is mild.

15.3.2.2   THE TREATMENT

The Modified Standard Drill is the initial drill of choice for patients who exhibit a partial response after the First Resistance Test and Second Resistance Test. In the first part of the drill, there is a reduction in intensity; one lens is worn at a time, and the other eye is not covered. Any drill performed without occluding an eye means that the wearing sequence starts with the weaker eye first. It sets the tone for the second part of the drill. Even though the patient covers one eye in the second part, the wearing sequence starts with the weaker eye. In the second part of the drill, there is an increase in stimulation; both lenses are worn together, and the other eye is covered to induce a multiplier effect. A multiplier effect is proposed here instead of the first part of the drill (in the Standard Drill). The increase in intensity is directed to the eyeball. (Refer to the chapter *Treating Mild and Moderate Myopia* for a description of the drill.)

After a few weeks, have the patient try the Modified Preliminary Drill. The eyeball can only retract so much when two lenses are worn for the Snellen Chart Drill in the second part of the Modified Standard Drill. The object of regard is only 5 ft away. The Modified Preliminary Drill just requires the patient to wear one lens for the Snellen Chart Drill. It projects the focal point farther from the retina. The Preliminary Drill also requires the patient to wear one lens for the Snellen Chart Drill, but it places more emphasis on the ciliary muscle rather than the rectus muscles. The Modified Preliminary Drill projects the focal point farther away since the Distance Drill only partially flattens the lens before engaging in the

Snellen Chart Drill. (Refer to the chapter *The Modified Preliminary Drill* for more information.)

There are certain extraneous variables that caused the ciliary muscles to partially spasm. Provide the patient with a list of possible factors that may contribute such an outcome. (Refer to the chapter *The Effort to See.*) Inform the patient about the different exercises and behavior changes (such as adjusting the distance for the reading range and midrange) to prevent near-point stress. When the patient is ready, determine the retention period. (Refer to the chapter *Wearing Schedule.*)

15.3.2.3   SECOND POSSIBLE RESPONSE FROM A PARTIAL RESISTANCE EYE

If the patient did not respond to the First Resistance Test, it is still possible to gain two or three lines after the Second Resistance Test. When that happens, it is still classified as a partial improvement. The depth perception is likely off. Although the patient sees line 8 on the Snellen chart, for example, the blurriness may start at line 5. A patient with a low resistance who sees line 8, the blurriness may start at line 8. Only line 8 is slightly blurred and line 7 is clear.

The first part of the Preliminary Drill was too intense even though it is a low resistance drill, but it responded to the second part of the Preliminary Drill (which is equivalent to the Second Resistance Test). The conditions of the Second Resistance Test allowed the ciliary muscle to relax partially. The decrease in stimulation to the ciliary muscle produced a corresponding change in the lens which in turn initiated a change in the eyeball. The lens needs to flatten first before the eyeball can change its shape.

15.3.2.4   THE TREATMENT

The Preliminary Drill is the initial drill of choice for patients who show no response to the First Resistance Test but became receptive to the Second Resistance Test and who experienced a two- or three-line improvement. The steps of the Preliminary Drill are the same as the steps for the First Resistance Test and the Second Resistance Test. After a few weeks, have the patient try the Modified Preliminary Drill. The Preliminary Drill is unstable since it mainly attends to the ciliary muscle. The eye can develop a resistance to the drill. The Modified Preliminary Drill entices the eyeball to reduce its myopic shape to alleviate the stress placed on the ciliary muscle.

There are certain extraneous variables that caused the ciliary muscles to partially spasm. Provide the patient with a list of possible factors that may contribute such an outcome. (Refer to the chapter *The Effort to See*.) Inform the patient about the different exercises and behavior changes (such as adjusting the distance for the reading range and midrange) to deal with the loss in depth perception. (Refer to the chapter *Treating a Loss of Depth Perception* for more information.) When the patient is ready, determine the retention period. (Refer to the chapter *Wearing Schedule*.)

15.3.3   THIRD RESISTANCE TEST

It is possible for the First Resistance Test and the Second Resistance Test to have no impact on the myopic eye. You have to move on to the next test, the Third Resistance Test. Steps 1 and 2 of the Standard Drill are equivalent to the Third Resistance Test. The multiplier effect increases the intensity of the drill to stimulate the eyeball to "shift." (Refer to the chapter *The Theory Behind the Standard Drill* for more information on the multiplier effect.)

The Third and Fourth Resistance Test are related. Together they are identical to Steps 1 to 4 of the Standard Drill. Once the patient begins the Third Resistance Test, instruct him to continue with the Fourth Resistance Test afterwards. It is as if he was performing the Standard Drill. If the eye is not responsive to the First and Second Resistance Test, it usually would not respond to the Third Resistance Test, but you still have to perform the test to set up the conditions for the Fourth Resistance Test. It is similar to how the First Resistance Test contributes to setting up the conditions for the Second Resistance Tests.

15.3.4   FOURTH RESISTANCE TEST

If there is no response to the First, Second, or Third Resistance Test, it may respond to the Fourth Resistance Test. Since the steps involved in the Fourth Resistance Test are the same as the Second Resistance Test, it poses the following question: Why can the Fourth Resistance Test unlock the partial spasm of the ciliary muscle and not the Second Resistance Test?

15.3.4.1   SETTING UP THE CONDITIONS

The difference between the Second Resistance Test and the Fourth Resistance Test is the influence from the previous test. The First and Third Resistance Tests set up certain conditions within the eye. The First Resistance Test prepares the eye for the Second Resistance Test in a different way. It mainly entices the ciliary muscle to relax in order to flatten the lens as much as possible. The Third Resistance test encourages the eyeball as well as the lens to participate in bringing a distant object into focus. It activates the lens to flatten less with the intention of enticing the eyeball to "shift" as much as possible. Although the patient does not see the improvement after the Third Resistance Test, it sets the stage for the Fourth Resistance Test by incrementally lowering the resistance of ciliary muscle. The eyeball may not actually "shift" until the Fourth Resistance Test.

15.3.4.2   THIRD POSSIBLE RESPONSE FROM A PARTIAL RESISTANCE EYE

The eye has to maintain the stimulation distributed to the ciliary muscle and rectus muscles before engaging in the Fourth Resistance Test. If the patient took too long performing the visual acuity test after the Third Resistance Test, it may interfere with the outcome from the Fourth Resistance Test (which is actually Steps 3 and 4 of the Standard Drill). In that case, start the Standard Drill over again from Step 1. (The patient is actually performing the Standard Drill from Steps 1 to 4.)

If the patient shows a partial response to the Fourth Resistance Test, the outcome would not be similar to the previous response after the Second Resistance Test. Instead of a three-line improvement on the Snellen chart, for example, there may only be a one-line improvement. It indicates that the crystalline lens is not as responsive.

15.3.4.3   THE TREATMENT

The Modified Standard Drill is the initial drill of choice for patients who exhibit a partial response after the Fourth Resistance Test. After performing the drill, there should be an improvement of another line or so if the ciliary muscle was not seized. Again, the eyeball can only retract so much with both lenses on in the second part of the Modified Standard Drill. The object of regard is only 5 ft away. After a few weeks, have the patient try the Modified Preliminary Drill. It projects the focal point farther from the retina to allow the eyeball to retract more.

There are certain extraneous variables that caused the ciliary muscles to tighten up in this manner such as developmental factors. (Refer to the chapter *Treating Progressive Myopia* for information on how myopia is different during development and postdevelopment.) Provide the patient with a list of other factors that contribute such an outcome. (Refer to the chapter *The Effort to See*.) Inform the patient about the different exercises and behavior changes (such as adjusting the distance for the reading range and midrange) to deal with the loss in depth perception. (Refer to the chapter *Treating a Loss of Depth Perception* for more information.) When the patient is ready, determine the retention period. (Refer to the chapter *Wearing Schedule*.)

15.4   TESTING THE RESISTANCE OF A SECONDARY REFRACTIVE ERROR

Although the resistance test are mainly intended for testing primary refractive errors, there are some exceptions. If the patient has a secondary refractive error, you are performing the resistance tests for a different reason. You are not trying to determine if the eye has a partial resistance. You already know there is a partial resistance when there is more than one refractive error (such as myopia and astigmatism). The compound astigmatic eye is likely to be within the myopic model if the sphere is mild or moderate. Instead you are relying on the tests to give you more information on borderline cases and to determine which drill is more effective. You are actually testing the level of astigmatism in the myopic eye.

15.4.1   TESTING MYOPIA AND ASTIGMATISM

You can apply the First Resistance Test to determine whether the Standard Drill or Modified Preliminary Drill is more effective to treat compound astigmatism when the cylinder is just at the threshold of what is considered high astigmatism. You want to know whether to treat the myopic or the astigmatic portion of the refractive error. You have to determine which feature represents the major problem.

If myopia is the major issue, the myopic eye would respond normally to the First Resistance Test. The minimal interference from astigmatism suggests applying the Standard Drill. If the interference is higher, the astigmatic eye would not response to the First Resistance Test. To rule out the possibility that you are treating an eye with a partial resistance, conduct the Second Resistance Test also. If the outcome is not satisfactory, it suggests applying the Modified Preliminary Drill. (Refer to the chapter *Case Examples* for more information.) Borderline cases are those where the cylinder reading is −1.00 D or when the cylinder is less than −1.00 D but equal to the sphere in mild cases of myopia. (Refer to the chapter *Treating Astigmatism* for more information.)

It should also be noted that the Third Resistance Test (which is actually the first part of the Standard Drill) may produce favorable results (at least temporarily) with borderline compound astigmatic cases after failing the first two tests. The improvement in visual acuity may even last for a month, but when the patient performs the drill again after the retention period, the eye may not respond to the drill. It is possible for the eye to build up a resistance against it. If the drill was too intense, it modified a part of the eye that did not need changing. After the First and Second Resistance Tests ruled out the possibility of applying the Standard Drill, continue with the Modified Preliminary Drill.

15.4.2   TESTING ANISOMETROPIA AND ASTIGMATISM

It is difficult to immediately determine whether astigmatism is predominant in an anisometopic eye with borderline astigmatism. Unlike compound myopia and borderline astigmatism, the compound anisometropic and astigmatic eye does not reject the First Resistance Test and Second Resistance Test right away even if the astigmatism is high. The anisometropia still responds to the test, but the high astigmatism will interferes with the outcome in a different way. The improvement may seem adequate at first; but if it was subjected to a load such as extensive work on the computer, the improvement may decrease after a few days.

If you treat it with the Modified Preliminary Drill, the retention period is much longer. An autorefractor reading would indicate that it reduces the sphere even though you are treating the astigmatism. Instead of testing for the resistance level of the astigmatism, just treat the compound anisometropic eye with the Modified Preliminary Drill. The patient would eventually have to perform the Modified Preliminary Drill anyway regardless if astigmatism or anisometropia is predominant.

A legitimate concern is in determining the wearing sequence in an eye with compound anisometropia, anisometropic amblyopia, and borderline astigmatism. Although the wearing sequence changes when applying the Modified Preliminary Drill in an eye with anisometropia and anisometropic amblyopia, the default is the normal wearing sequence when the astigmatism is high. Even if the astigmatism is borderline, in most cases the patient would begin the Modified Preliminary Drill with the weaker eye first.

15.5   THE RESISTANCE TESTS

The steps for the different tests are as follows:

15.5.1   FIRST RESISTANCE TEST

1. Wear the lens on the *weaker eye* only. Look outside at an object about 500 or 1000 ft away. (Look 500 ft away if you have moderate myopia. Look 1000 ft away if you have mild myopia.) **Do not cover** the other eye that does not have the lens on. Keep both eyes open. Do the Distance Drill for 30 s. Then take the lens off.
2. Test the patient's visual acuity.
3. Wear the lens on the *better eye* only. Look at an object about 500 or 1000 ft away. **Do not cover** the other eye. Keep both eyes open. Do the Distance Drill for 30 s. Then take the lens off.
4. Test the patient's visual acuity.

15.5.2   SECOND RESISTANCE TEST (TO BE PERFORMED IMMEDIATELY AFTER THE FIRST RESISTANCE TEST)

1. Wear the lens on the *weaker eye* only. Perform the Snellen Chart Drill with the *weaker eye* first. **Cover** the other eye. Hold the palm about 2–3 in. from the eye. Keep both eyes open. Stand 5 ft away from the chart. Read line 7 at a rate of 1 s per letter for five times. Then take the lens off.
2. Test the patient's visual acuity.

3. Wear the lens on the *better eye* only. Perform the Snellen Chart Drill with the *better eye*. **Cover** the other eye. Hold the palm about 2–3 in. from the eye. Keep both eyes open. Stand 5.0 ft away from the chart. Read line 7 at a rate of 1 s per letter five times. Then take the lens off.
4. Test the patient's visual acuity.

15.5.3 THIRD RESISTANCE TEST

1. Wear both lenses. Look outside at an object about 500 or 1000 ft away with the *better eye*. (Look 500 ft away if you have moderate myopia. Look 1000 ft away if you have mild myopia.) **Cover** the other eye. Hold the palm 2–3 in. from the eye to prevent instrument myopia. Keep both eyes open. Do the Distance drill for 30 s.
2. With both lenses still on, look at an object about 500 or 1000 ft away with the *weaker eye*. **Cover** the other eye. Hold the palm 2–3 in. from the eye. Keep both eyes open. Do the Distance Drill for 30 s. Then take both lenses off.
3. Test the patient's visual acuity.

15.5.4 FOURTH RESISTANCE TEST (TO BE DONE IMMEDIATELY AFTER THE THIRD RESISTANCE TEST)

1. Wear the lens on the *better eye* only. Perform the Snellen Chart Drill with the *better eye* first. **Cover** the other eye. Hold the palm two to three in. from the eye. Keep both eyes open. Stand 5 ft away from the chart. Read line 7 at a rate of 1 s per letter for five times. Then take the lens off.
2. Test the patient's visual acuity.
3. Wear the lens on the *weaker eye* only. Perform the Snellen Chart Drill with the *weaker eye*. **Cover** the other eye. Hold the palm 2–3 in. from the eye. Keep both eyes open. Stand 5.0 ft away from the chart. Read line 7 at a rate of 1 s per letter. Read that line five times. Then take the lens off.
4. Test the patient's visual acuity.

KEYWORDS

- first resistance test
- second resistance test
- third resistance test
- fourth resistance test
- low resistance
- partial resistance
- high resistance

CHAPTER 16

THE THEORY BEHIND THE STANDARD DRILL

ABSTRACT

The Standard Drill represents one of my inventions: the multiplier effect. The multiplier effect flattens the lens and eyeball as much as possible in the first part of the drill before resorting to the indirect effect in the second part of the drill to flatten the eyeball some more. It is designed to treat a primary refractive error. The moderate myopic eye can take the drill's high intensity due to the features of a primary refractive error. It is in the −0.75 D to −1.75 D range. The prescription for both eyes is the same or with a disparity of −0.25 D or less.

I also came up with a variation of the multiplier effect to deal with secondary refractive errors such as anisometropia and compound astigmatism: the indirect effect. It was like an invention within an invention. The indirect effect, or indirect influence as I sometimes called it, is a partial multiplier effect.

The multiplier effect can be thought of as a more intense indirect effect. Going by that definition, the Standard Drill is the most intense drill. The intensity of a drill is not positively correlated to the degree of improvement. A flexible ciliary muscle allows for a high intensity drill, but a ciliary muscle that is less flexible due to a partial spasticity requires a less intense drill. The type of refractive error also needs to be taken into account. The presence of astigmatism, for example, introduces another refractive error on top of myopia. The partial resistance requires another drill with a lower intensity factor. A decrease in intensity allows the motor cortex to manipulate a specific meridian of the crystalline lens instead of the whole lens.

Similar to the Preliminary Drill, the Standard Drill consists of the Distance Drill and the Snellen Chart Drill. The patient would perform the Distance Drill in the first part of the Standard Drill, and the Snellen Chart

Drill in the second part, and then the Distance Drill again in the third part without wearing any ortho C lens. (Refer to the chapter *What do Do* for a description of how to perform the supplementary drills.)

16.1   THE STANDARD DRILL'S ROLE IN THE TREATMENT FOR MYOPIA

16.1.1   BOTH EYES EQUAL OR WITH A DISPARITY OF −0.25 D

If the prescription for each eye is the same or if the difference between them is −0.25 D, then the flatness factor is equal to the absolute value of the prescription for each eye. These conditions offer the best improvement in visual acuity and retention after performing the Standard Drill. It allows the multiplier effect to take place without creating an overcorrection.

16.1.2   WHY A MAXIMUM IMPROVEMENT IN VISUAL ACUITY AND RETENTION

There is a maximum improvement in visual acuity and retention due to the following:

- A primary refractive error allows for a multiplier effect.
- A low disparity in prescription between each eye.
- Mild or moderate myopia inherited less extraneous variables.
- The myopia of both eyes fall within the myopic model.
- There is a low resistance (to ortho C).
- The lens and eyeball became myopic in the right proportion.

16.1.3   INCREASE IN VISUAL ACUITY

After performing the Standard Drill, the first thing that is noticeable is the immediate increase in visual acuity. There is a maximum reversal in the myopic shape of the lens and eyeball due to the multiplier effect. I had one participant who was so excited after just the first application that he emailed to me a description of what he could see the next day. His prescription prior to the treatment was OD −1.50 D and OS −1.75 D. His office was illuminated only by artificial light, but he could see letters equal to the size of the 20/15 line on the Snellen chart at 12–13 ft away without much effort. He also maintained the improvement for over a month before he felt the need to wear the ortho C lens again.

16.1.4   INCREASE IN RETENTION

16.1.4.1   A FLATTER NEUTRAL SHAPE OF THE LENS

The maximum reversal in the myopic shape of the lens and eyeball in the right proportion also contributes to an increase in retention. The Standard Drill flattens the crystalline lens' occluded neutral shape by a multiple of the contact lens's base curve, and that induces a reduction in the elongated eyeball in the right proportion. The phenomenon can be demonstrated by treating the moderate myopic eye with just the first part of the Preliminary Drill and comparing the outcome to just the first part of the Standard Drill. By keeping both eyes opened in the first part of the Preliminary Drill, the occluded neutral shape of the eye was not activated.

By just flattening the lens' open neutral shape, you are not flattening its maximum bulged shape. The lens already assumed a flatter shape even before performing the first part of the Preliminary Drill. There is some free play within the restriction imposed by the tension of the oblique muscles. It allows the lens to bulge for close work and to partially flatten for the distance. You have to expose the lens' occluded neutral shape instead of its open neutral shape. It is its occluded neutral shape that became myopic. Its focal point is farther from the retina. When the lens flatten during the first part of the Standard Drill, there is still a gap to allow the myopic eyeball to retract.

If you test the patient's visual acuity in a dim room on a projected eye chart after performing the first part of the Preliminary Drill, the outcome is less than the reading obtained in a well-lit room—especially if the eye chart was by a source of natural light. It is comparable to the effect natural relaxation exercises have on the crystalline lens. If the occluded neutral shape of the crystalline lens does not flatten sufficiently, the sclera would not participate in the reversal process. A conventional eye exam cannot pick up the improvement experienced by the patient since the crystalline lens' open neutral shape was bypassed. The eyeball remain myopic.

How do you expose the lens' occluded neutral shape? The patient cannot perform the drill at night. It would not work. It lacks a "focal point draw." All the drills need to be performed during the day. To expose the lens' occluded neutral shape, cover the other eye. When it bulges more in the occluded eye, the lens also assumes a bulged shape in the open eye. There is more room for the lens to reverse; and that stimulates the eyeball to participate in the process.

If you apply the Preliminary Drill as whole to treat a primary refractive error, the results would still be unstable. The multiplier effect was not included in the first part of the drill to encourage the eyeball to retract. The eye's reversal in the second part of the Preliminary Drill is insufficient to alleviate the stress from day to day work imposed on the crystalline lens. Then again, the Preliminary Drill was meant to treat a different problem. Its flatness factor was mainly designed to address the excess tension of the ciliary muscle of an anisometropic eye without excessively altering the lens' occluded neutral shape in the better eye (since the contact lens' flatness factor was determined by the higher myopic eye). You need the proper drill to treat a specific problem.

16.2   APPLICATION OF THE DRILL IN THE TREATMENT FOR MYOPIA

16.2.1   FIRST PART OF THE DRILL

16.2.1.1   STEP 1

16.2.1.1.1   The Direct Influence on the Opened Better Eye

Both lenses are worn in the first part of the drill. In Step 1, the patient performs the Distance Drill with the better eye first. Although the prescription is the same, you determine the weaker eye by conducting a Visual Acuity Test. Refer to the section *Determining the Weaker Eye* in *The Procedure*. The direct influence of the better eye also improves the visual acuity of the weaker eye. The weaker eye benefits from the indirect effect. However, there is a tradeoff. Wearing a contact lens on the better eye first means that the crystalline lens tends to "shift" more. It has a lower resistance. It can close the gap between the focal point and the retina and not leave enough room for the eyeball to flatten.

To increase the gap between the focal point and the retina, the other eye is covered to expose the lens' occluded neutral shape (in the open eye as well as the occluded eye). To prevent the aperture from closing too much, remind the patient to remain inside the dwelling and look outside while performing the Distance Drill. It also helps to stand a few feet away from the window ledge.

You want to flatten the lens' occluded neutral shape first to activate the eyeball to change its curvature for distant focusing. The lens' occluded neutral shape needs to be flattened first before the eyeball can flatten. The retraction of the eyeball in the first part of the drill reduces how much it needs to "shift" later.

16.2.1.1.2   The Multiplier Effect on the Covered Weaker Eye

When the occluded eye receives the indirect influence from the lens on the opened better eye in Step 1, the ortho C lens on the weaker eye does something with the message to increase the stimulation on the weaker eye even though that eye is covered. The first multiplier effect occurs when the lens amplifies the indirect effect. The indirect influence stimulates the ciliary muscle to relax. The lens' occluded neutral shape would flatten out. It is its occluded neutral shape that changes instead of the open neutral shape because the eye was occluded. It flattened out indirectly via the relaxed oblique muscles from the other eye instead of a "focal point draw." The lens' occluded neutral shape was manipulated indirectly.

The rectus muscles would participate in the reversal process by tightening up to reduce the elongated sclera. The gap between the focal point and the retina of the open eye neurologically determines how much the sclera of the occluded eye retracts. The "contact lens draw" from the ortho C lens on the occluded eye may amplify the indirect influence. Thus the sclera retracts due to a multiplier effect.

16.2.1.1.3   The Multiplier Effect on the Open Better Eye

At the same time, the weaker occluded eye induces an indirect effect on the opened better eye in Step 1. The indirect influence relayed is actually the multiplier effect from the occluded eye. Although the better eye was not occluded, the indirect effect bypasses the crystalline lens. There is no interference from a negative tear layer. The indirect influence was from an eye that was occluded—not from a contact lens. It allowed the transference of a shortened eyeball. The "contact lens draw" from the ortho C lens on the open eye may amplify the indirect influence. Thus the sclera retracts due to a second multiplier effect. If you took a visual acuity test after your patient conducts the Distance Drill in Step 1 of the Standard Drill, you would usually find the better and weaker eye improved equally and by the same amount. It is an indication that the multiplier effect improved both the occluded eye and the open eye.

16.2.1.2   STEP 2

When the patient wears the lens on the weaker eye in Step 2, the process starts all over again. If you took another visual acuity test after your patient performs the Distant Drill in Step 2 with the weaker eye, you may find that the better eye (which was occluded) sees slightly better because it has a lower resistance in terms of having a lower prescription. It is an indication that the multiplier effect further improved the occluded eye.

16.2.2   THE SECOND PART OF THE DRILL

The lens is worn one at a time in the second part of the drill. Unlike the first part of the drill, there is no contact lens on the covered eye to create a multiplier effect. It would be too intense to introduce a multiplier effect when the object of regard is 5 ft away. The indirect effect on the occluded eye is not amplified. The conditions allowing the eyeball to flatten further in the second part of the drill are the same as in the second part of the Preliminary Drill. The influence from the ortho C lens in the second part of the Standard Drill is similar to the influence in the second part of the Preliminary Drill.

The improvement in visual acuity in the second part of the Standard Drill is on top of the improvement from the multiplier effect in the first part of the drill. The patient would wear one lens at a time starting with the better eye first. Attending to the better eye first in Step 3 is different from the wearing sequence in the Preliminary Drill. It is the wearing sequence in the first part of the specific drill that determines the wearing sequence in the second part.

Usually, the patient would gain two lines on the Snellen eye chart after the first part of the Standard Drill and another line after the second part. Omitting the second part of the Standard Drill may not maximize the reinforcement in retention. The further reduction in the myopic shape of the eyeball in the second part of the drill contributes to the increase in visual acuity and retention.

16.2.2.1   Why Flatten the Lens in the First Part of the Drill as much as Possible?

If the myopic occluded neutral shape of the lens was not flattened as much as possible in the first part of the drill, it would be flattened further in the second part of the drill. In the second part, the object of regard is only 5 ft away. The gap between the focal point and the retina poses a restriction on how much it can flatten. It was not meant to flatten the lens extensively. The setting was designed to entice the occluded shape of the lens to flatten slightly in order to entice the eyeball to also flatten slightly. The eyeball retracts slightly to alleviate the increase in effort to bring an object into focus under less than optimum conditions. The overall improvement sets the stage for the third part of the drill.

16.3.1   THE THIRD PART OF THE DRILL

Fusion refers to the synchronization between the lens and eyeball. In step 5, the patient would perform the Distance Drill without wearing any lenses. The same object of regard in Step 1 is sought out instead of referring to another object closer or farther away. You want the crystalline lens to readjust. It did not flatten out sufficiently in the second part of the drill (since the object of regard is only 5 ft away). It must flatten as much as possible again for the distance given the renewed shape of the eyeball. The oblique muscles still retain the relaxation from the "contact lens draw" long enough to allow a final adjustment between the ciliary muscle and oblique muscles before the tension of the intraocular and extraocular muscles settles. Most patients notice a further enhancement in visual acuity after the last step.

16.3.1.1   THE STANDARD DRILL TO TREAT MILD AND MODERATE MYOPIA FROM −0.75 D TO −1.75 D

1.   Wear both lenses. Look outside at an object about 500 or 1000 ft away with the *better eye*. (Look 500 ft away if you have moderate myopia. Look 1000 ft away if you have mild myopia.) **Cover** the other eye. Hold the palm 2–3 in. from the eye to prevent instrument myopia. Keep both eyes open. Do the Distance drill for 30 s.

2. With both lenses still on, look at an object about 500 or 1000 ft away with the *weaker eye*. **Cover** the other eye. Look at the same object in Step 1. Hold the palm 2–3 in. from the eye. Keep both eyes open. Do the Distance Drill for 30 s. Then take off the lens on the weaker eye.

3. With only the lens on the *better eye*, perform the Snellen Chart Drill. **Cover** the other eye. Hold the palm 2–3 in. from the eye. Keep both eyes open. Stand 5.0 ft away from the chart. Read line 7 five times at a rate of 1 s per letter. Then take the lens off.

4. Insert the lens on the *weaker eye* and perform the Snellen Chart Drill. **Cover** the other eye. Hold the palm 2–3 in. from the eye. Keep both eyes open. Stand 5.0 ft away from the chart. Read line 7 five times at a rate of 1 s per letter. Then take the lens off.

5. *Without* any lenses on, look outside at an object about 500 or 1000 ft away with *both* eyes. Look at the same object in Step 1. Do the Distance Drill for 1 min with both eyes. **Not** with each eye separately.

KEYWORDS

- **the theory behind the Standard Drill**
- **multiplier effect**
- **Standard Drill**
- **direct influence**
- **indirect influence**
- **lens' occluded neutral shape**
- **fusion**

CHAPTER 17

THE THEORY BEHIND THE PRELIMINARY DRILL

ABSTRACT

Sometimes the patient performs the Preliminary Drill first before the Modified Preliminary Drill during the treatment for anisometropia. The conventional definition for anisometropia is a difference of -1.00 D between the right and left eye. In reference to what can be treated by ortho C, a disparity of -0.75 also qualifies as anisometropia. The weaker eye predetermines the flatness factor for both lenses. The treatable range is when one eye is moderate (from -1.00 D to -1.75 D) and the other is in the midrange (from -2.00 D to -2.75 D). The treatment is optimal when the better eye is -1.00 D to -1.25 D, and the weaker eye is -2.00 D or -2.25 D. The patient needs to realize that the Preliminary Drill is temporary. It is usually performed first to prepare the eye for the Modified Preliminary Drill. You eventually have to treat anisometropia with the Modified Preliminary Drill.

According to research, the myopic shape of the crystalline lens and eyeball is not in proportion to the thickness of the ciliary muscle (Kuchem et al., 2013). The increase in tension of the ciliary muscle of the weaker eye due to near-point stress spills over onto the better eye. The ciliary muscle of the better eye neurologically inherits the same thickness. The myopic shape of the crystalline lens and eyeball of the better eye, however, is not in proportion to the thickness of the ciliary muscle.

It is better for a less intense drill (i.e., the Preliminary Drill) to relax the ciliary muscle rather than a more intense drill (i.e., the Standard Drill). The Preliminary Drill relaxes the ciliary muscle of the better eye without overcorrecting the lens or the axial length of the eyeball. Once you attend to the ciliary muscle before increasing the tension of the rectus muscles, the Modified Preliminary Drill becomes more effective when it attends to the eyeball as well as the crystalline lens.

17.1　OTHER REASONS FOR ADOPTING THE PRELIMINARY DRILL FIRST

I called the initial drill the Preliminary Drill since the patient performs it first before the Modified Preliminary Drill—and sometimes even before the Standard Drill. It does not interfere with the application of those drills. Before I elaborate on how the Preliminary Drill contributes to the treatment for anisometropia, the following are some other reasons why the patient may perform the drill first.

17.1.1　WEARING SEQUENCE TEST

The Preliminary Drill is part of the Wearing Sequence Test. The first part of the Preliminary Drill is equivalent to the steps in the Wearing Sequence Test. The patient must perform that test prior to any drill to determine which lens to wear first or which eye to perform the drill first.

17.1.2　RESISTANCE TESTS

The first and second parts of the Preliminary Drill are also equivalent to the First Resistance Test and Second Resistance Test. Those tests determine the resistance of the eye. When the patient performs the Wearing Sequence Test, you are also considering the response to the First Resistance Test at the same time. To complete the Second Resistance Test, the patient is actually completing the second part of the Preliminary Drill. (Refer to the chapter *The Procedure* for the context surrounding the tests.)

17.1.3　IN CASE OF AN ERROR

It is easier to correct a mistake while practicing with the Preliminary Drill compared with the Standard Drill. The latter drill prolongs the change in visual acuity by setting up a higher resistance to stress from working in the near, intermediate, and distant ranges (without glasses) compared to the Preliminary Drill. In that respect, if a mistake was made (such as mixing up the lenses), it is harder to correct the relapse in visual acuity after the multiplier effect reinforces the incorrect neurological message.

17.1.4   FIRST TIME WEARERS

The Preliminary Drill is beneficial for patients who are sensitive to wearing a rigid contact lens. The Standard Drill requires wearing both lenses in Steps 1 and 2. Having both lenses on can be challenging for someone who never worn contact lenses before. It is irritating to have a foreign object on the cornea, and the tearing may interfere with the "contact lens draw" and "focal point draw." Wearing the lenses one at a time reduces the discomfort from having something in both eyes for the first time. The patient can practice with the Preliminary Drill to adapt to the contact lens before attempting the Standard Drill.

The improvement in visual acuity after performing the Preliminary Drill tends to fluctuate if the required drill is the Standard Drill. The patient would have to switch over to the Standard Drill after about 2 weeks to avoid incurring an excessive "effort to see." Otherwise, there is the tendency for a resistance to build up against the drill if the patient constantly makes an excessive "effort to see" under less than favorable conditions. On the other hand, if the patient has worn contact lenses before or if there is no problem adapting to them after performing the different resistance tests, then you might consider assigning the Standard Drill afterwards. (Yes, adapting to the discomfort can be that quick.)

17.2   THE PRELIMINARY DRILL'S ROLE IN THE TREATMENT FOR ANISOMETROPIA

17.2.1   PREPARING THE EYE FOR THE MODIFIED PRELIMINARY DRILL

The Preliminary Drill's role is mainly to lower the spasticity of the ciliary muscle without overcorrecting the eyeball. The drill prepares the eye for the Modified Preliminary Drill which attends to both the shape of the lens and eyeball of an anisometropic eye. Its deviation eye is different. It is not just a matter of attending to the myopic shape of the lens or eyeball but also to the spasticity of the ciliary muscle. According to Kuchem et al. (2013), the better eye has the same ciliary muscle thickness as the higher myopic eye with a longer axial length. The axial length of the better eye is less. Thus, the ciliary spasm of the better eye is high while the deviation of the eyeball is less in proportion.

The problem is not just related to near-point stress. The increase in tension of the ciliary muscle of the weaker eye due to near-point stress spilled over onto the better eye. The ciliary muscle of the better eye neurologically inherits the same thickness. The myopic shape of the crystalline lens and eyeball of the better eye, however, is not in proportion to the thickness of the ciliary muscle. It is better for a less intense drill (i.e., the Preliminary Drill) to relax the ciliary muscle rather than a more intense drill (i.e., the Standard Drill). A multiplier effect would overcorrect the eyeball in the better eye. It deviated less than the weaker eye.

The Preliminary Drill tends to bypass the eyeball and overcorrect the lens, but it is better to overcorrect the crystalline lens than the eyeball. The patient can experience the overcorrection after the first application. It is not unusual to have a four-line improvement or more on the Snellen chart. The patient would experience it with both eyes. The improvement is mainly noticeable outdoors during the day, but it suffers a bit indoors under dim or artificial lighting and at night since the eyeball did not follow suit.

It is possible to immediately perform the Modified Preliminary Drill without resorting to the Preliminary Drill if the better eye is within the optimal range. It depends on the extent of the ciliary muscle spasm. It is different from the spasm directly induced by a minus lens. The spasm in the better eye was indirectly induced by the weaker eye. So, if you had the patient try the Modified Preliminary Drill first and if you found that there could be more room for improvement, then have him try the Preliminary Drill. The Preliminary Drill focuses mainly on the ciliary muscle. If the results are favorable, then continue the drill for a couple of weeks before attempting the Modified Preliminary Drill again.

17.2.2   THE DILEMMA

Unlike treating mild or moderate myopia without a disparity in prescription, you cannot match the flatness factor to the prescription of each eye. The flatness factor for an anisometropic eye depends on the prescription of the weaker eye. It is the determining factor for the flatness of both lenses. Consider the following prescription: OD -1.00 D and OS -2.50 D. You need a flatness factor of 2.0 D for the better eye as well as the weaker eye to relieve the tension of the ciliary muscle by that amount; the tension of the ciliary muscle in the better eye is the same as the weaker eye. If the prescription of the weaker eye is over -2.00 D, the flatness factor is still

2.0 D. It is the maximum recommended flatness to treat anisometropia when the weaker eye is in the midrange. When you design both lenses with a flatness factor of 2.0 D to address the tension, however, it poses the following dilemma:

- The lens' flatness factor for the better eye correctly offsets the tension of the oblique muscles (and thus the ciliary muscle) but it does not correspond to its refractive error. In the above example, it is −1.00 D despite the excessive spasm of the ciliary muscle. Assigning a flatness factor of 2.0 D can create an overcorrection.
- There is the risk that the ciliary muscle of the better eye may tighten up some more due to the tear factor. It would have a negative direct effect on the crystalline lens before the "contact lens draw" can entice the ciliary muscle to respond to the reduction in the tension of the oblique muscles. Due to the flatness of the contact lens, it would be as if though the patient was wearing a high minus lens.
- The maximum flatness of an ortho C lens is 1.75 D if the prescription is in the moderate range. Wearing a lens flatter than 1.75 D would tend to induce ortho K by pushing against the cornea instead of "drawing" on it when the contact lens solution drains and reduces the meniscus. Ortho C and ortho K do not mix.

17.2.3 DEALING WITH THE DILEMMA

The Preliminary Drill deals with the dilemma as follows:

- Both eyes were kept opened in Steps 1 and 2. The occluded neutral shape of the eye was not activated. By flattening the lens' open neutral shape, its free play is included to minimize how much the lens' occluded neutral shape can flatten—and thus how much the eyeball flattens.
- The contact lens is worn on the weaker eye first in Steps 1 to activate an indirect instead of a direct influence on the better eye. By flattening the crystalline lens slightly, the better eye temporarily increases its resistance against a negative tear layer from a flatter contact lens.
- Stand a few feet away from the window sill.
- Perform the drill on a cloudy day to avoid a direct glare from the sun.

- The contact lens is worn for only 15 s in Steps 1 and 2.

17.3 APPLICATION OF THE DRILL IN THE TREATMENT FOR ANISOMETROPIA

The steps of the Preliminary Drill are identical to the First Resistance Test and Second Resistance Test. The drill determines the flexibility of the ciliary muscle and how much the lens can flatten. It offers a hint at how much the eyeball elongated and thus, how much it needs to flatten.

For example, if there is a three-line improvement after performing Steps 1 and 2 of the Preliminary Drill, then you know that the eyeball only deviated partially. The lens was capable of assuming an excessive bulged shape. Since most of the deviation is in the lens, the eyeball did not have to elongate that much to alleviate near-point stress. The patient would probably gain another line after performing Steps 3 and 4. Even though the visual acuity is extremely sharp during the day, nighttime visual acuity may be a bit off. Thus, the patient needs to perform the Modified Preliminary Drill to "shift" the eyeball a bit more. The Preliminary Drill was still too intense for the ciliary muscle. The lens flattened too much to allow enough room for the eye to retract.

17.3.1   THE FIRST PART OF THE DRILL

17.3.1.1   STEP 1

17.3.1.1.1   The Distance Drill's Effect on the Weaker Eye

The patient performs the Distance Drill in Step 1 by wearing the lens on the weaker eye. The "contact lens draw" induces a direct influence. The "loosening" of the oblique muscles by 2.0 D improves the shape of the crystalline lens.

17.3.1.1.2   The Distance Drill's Effect on the Better Eye

The Distance Drill in Step 1 also stimulates the ciliary muscle of the better eye to relax indirectly and thus induce a flatter crystalline lens. It allows the "contact lens draw" on the weaker eye to indirectly influence the oblique muscles of the better eye without simultaneously creating a minus tear layer. The crystalline lens of the better eye flattens in the same proportion as how much it bulged due to the tension of the ciliary muscle.

17.3.1.2   STEP 2

The patient performs the Distance Drill in Step 2 by wearing the lens on the better eye. The flatness factor is 2.0 D. If the prescription of the better eye was -1.00 D, the lens exceeded the maximum flatness for that eye by 1.00 D. The negative tear layer tends to overcorrect the crystalline lens first before the ortho C lens can attend to the tension of the oblique muscles.

However, the indirect influence on the better eye in Step 1 flattens the crystalline lens to insulate it from the direct influence of a flatter lens for that eye in Step 2. The new shape momentarily resists the impact from a negative tear layer. It takes a bit longer to entice the lens to bulge. To further minimize the risk of inducing the lens to bulge, the wearing time is 15 s; and both eyes were opened to expose the crystalline lens' open neutral shape.

17.3.2   THE SECOND PART OF THE DRILL

17.3.2.1   STEP 3

17.3.2.1.1   The Snellen Chart Drill's Effect on the Weaker Eye

The dilemma becomes more pronounce in the second part of the drill. It is performed 5 ft away from the object of regard. At that distance, the eye converges slightly. The inward pull of the medial rectus muscle assists the eyeball to retract once the "contact lens draw" "loosens" the oblique muscles.

At 5 ft from the Snellen chart, however, a flatter lens on the better eye may entice the crystalline lens to flatten excessively. To deal with the dilemma, the lens is worn on the weaker eye first in Step 3. The wearing sequence of the second part of the drill is the same as the first part. The patient exposes the occluded neutral shape of the lens by occluding the other eye without the contact lens on. By covering one eye, the crystalline lens takes on an occluded neutral myopic shape in the opened eye as well as in the covered eye. Monocular vision is more challenging for the myopic eye compared to the emmetropic eye. The lens in its occluded neutral shape bulges more compared to its open neutral shape. To make it more challenging, the Snellen chart is hung in artificial light. The aperture of the eye opens more.

Those conditions displace the focal point farther from the retina to allow enough room for the sclera to "shift." The lens would not flatten as much as in the first part of the drill. The restrictions imposed on how much the lens can flatten causes the eyeball to flatten to alleviate the excess effort. It is the reverse of near-point stress.

17.3.2.1.2   The Snellen Chart Drill's Effect on the Better Eye

The indirect influence relaxes the tension of the oblique muscles of the better eye. The lens and eyeball are not overcorrected. The motor cortex differentiates the deviation between the better eye and weaker eye. Despite the increase in tension of the oblique muscles, it corrects the better eye in the proper proportion—in the same proportion as how much it deviated.

17.3.2.2   STEP 4

The flatter crystalline lens from part 1 of the drill still insulates the better eye from the direct influence of a contact lens with a flatness factor of 2.0 D in Step 4. The eye is subjected to the same conditions as in Step 3. Thus, the better eye becomes receptive to a flatter contact lens. The result from the direct influence in Step 4 completes the total effect on the better eye. It is on top of the benefit gained from the indirect influences from Steps 1 and 3 and the direct influence from Step 2. It is the combined benefits from those steps that stimulate the better eye to gain maximum improvement.

The better eye transmits an indirect total influence to the weaker eye. The result from the indirect influence from Step 4 completes the total effect on the weaker eye. It is on top of the benefit gained from the direct influences from Steps 1 and 3 and from the indirect influence from Step 2. It is the combined benefits from those Steps that stimulate the weaker eye to gain maximum improvement.

Finishing with the lens in the better eye sets the standard in the patient's binocular visual acuity. The binocular vision of a myopee takes on the visual acuity of the better eye. Ortho C takes advantage of this phenomenon. Even if there is still a bit of disparity between the right and left eye afterwards, the better eye tends to bring distant objects into focus, and the weaker eye tends to bring near and intermediate objects into focus. A variation of monovision is at work. (Refer to the chapter *Treating Anisometropia* for more information on monovision.)

It is not that effective if you started off by having the patient wear the ortho C lens in the better eye first in Step 1. Going by this sequence, you would finish off with a total direct influence on the weaker eye. Your binocular visual acuity would then take on the features of the weaker eye.

17.3.3   THE THIRD PART OF THE DRILL

17.3.3.1   FUSION

Step 5 of the Standard Drill is not included in the Preliminary Drill. Most anisometropic and astigmatic participants ended up seeing worse when attempting this step with both eyes together. In order for fusion to take place, it is not just a matter of synchronizing the lens and eyeball of each eye but also the right and left eye. Step 5 of the Standard Drill seems to favor the former more than the latter when performing it with both eyes open. It also tends to stimulate the better eye more than the weaker eye. The third part of the Preliminary Drill, Steps 5 and 6, attempts to synchronize the right and left eye as well as the lens and eyeball of each eye.

17.3.3.2   READJUSTING THE LENS TO TAKE INTO ACCOUNT THE REDUCTION OF THE ELONGATED EYE

The patient has to perform Steps 5 and 6 to readjust the lens' occluded neutral shape to take into account the reduction in the eye's elongated shape in Steps 3 and 4. The adjustment is made by performing the Distance Drill with each eye without any lens on starting with the weaker eye. When switching over to the Modified Preliminary Drill, it includes these steps only in the treatment for simple astigmatism or compound myopia and high astigmatism. It omits these steps in the treatment for anisometropia, compound anisometropia and high astigmatism, and compound anisometropia and amblyopia.

17.4   THE PRELIMINARY DRILL TO TREAT ANISOMETROPIA

1. Wear the lens on the *weaker eye* only. Look outside at an object about 500 ft away. **Do not cover** the other eye. Keep both eyes open. Do the Distance Drill for 15 s. Then take the lens off.
2. Wear the lens on the *better eye* only. Look outside at an object about 500 ft away. **Do not cover** the other eye. Look at the same object in Step 1. Keep both eyes open. Do the Distance Drill for 15 s. Then take the lens off.
3. Wear the lens on the *weaker eye* only. Perform the Snellen Chart Drill with the *weaker eye* first. **Cover** the other eye. Hold the palm about 2–3 in. from the eye. Keep both eyes open. Stand 5.0 ft away from the chart. Read line 7 five times at a rate of 1 s per letter. Then take the lens off.
4. Wear the lens on the *better eye* only. Perform the Snellen Chart Drill with the *better eye*. **Cover** the other eye. Hold the palm about 2–3 in. from the eye. Keep both eyes open. Stand 5.0 ft away from the chart. Read line 7 five times at a rate of 1 s per letter. Then take the lens off.
5. Without any lens on, look outside at an object about 500 ft away with the *weaker eye.* **Cover** the other eye. Look at the same object in Step 1. Leave a slight gap 2–3 in. from the eye. Keep both eyes open. Do the Distance Drill for 30 s.
6. Without any lens on, look outside at an object about 500 ft away with the *better eye.* **Cover** the other eye. Look at the same object in Step 1. Leave a slight gap 2–3 in. from the eye. Keep both eyes open. Do the Distance Drill for 30 s.

KEYWORDS

- **indirect effect**
- **Preliminary Drill**
- **Modified Preliminary Drill**
- **anisometropia**
- **ciliary muscle thickness**
- **ciliary muscle spasm**
- **axial length**

CHAPTER 18

THE THEORY BEHIND THE MODIFIED PRELIMINARY DRILL

ABSTRACT

The Modified Preliminary Drill represents my other inventions: the indirect effect (Yee, 2011). The Modified Preliminary Drill is a variation of the Preliminary Drill. You will apply it more frequently than the Standard Drill to treat various types of secondary refractive errors. I designed it to treat anisometropia, simple astigmatism, and "compound astigmatism" (or compound myopia and astigmatism). It is the decrease in the Modified Preliminary Drill's intensity compared to the other drills that make it appropriate in the treatment for secondary refractive errors. The correct intensity influences the crystalline lens to flatten just the right amount to cause the eyeball to retract. If the crystalline lens flattens excessively, the eyeball cannot respond properly.

To treat anisometropia, you do not have to abide by its classical definition: a disparity of −1.0 D between the right and left eye. If the disparity is −0.75 D, you can still treat it as anisometropia by following the same protocol. (Refer to the chapter *Treating Anisometropia* for more information.) Although a disparity of −0.50 D does not qualify as anisometropia, you can still immediately treat it by applying the Modified Preliminary Drill without starting with the Preliminary Drill. (Refer to the chapter *Treating Mild and Moderate Myopia* for more information.) To treat astigmatism, it can take the form of simple astigmatism, or it can be combined with myopia, anisometropia, or even anisometropic amblyopia. (Refer to the chapter *Treating Astigmatism* for more information.)

18.1 INTENSITY FACTOR

It is the decrease in the Modified Preliminary Drill's intensity compared to the other drills that makes it appropriate in the treatment for secondary refractive errors mentioned in this book. After performing the Modified Preliminary Drill, the direct and indirect effects from each supplementary drill are inline (as shown in Table 18.1). After performing the Standard or Preliminary Drill, the direct and indirect effects from each supplementary drill are alternating (as shown in Table 18.2). An alternating arrangement is more intense. The Modified Preliminary Drill is less intense than the Preliminary Drill or Standard Drill. The ranking of the main drills in terms of their order of intensity from the least intense to the most intense is as follows: the Modified Preliminary Drill, the Preliminary Drill, and the Standard Drill.

18.2   INLINE DIRECT AND INDIRECT EFFECT

Table 18.1 represents the arrangement of the direct and indirect effects after performing the Modified Preliminary Drill. Suppose the wearing sequence starts with the right eye. The patient performs the Distance Drill in Step 1 and the Snellen Chart Drill in Step 2 with the right eye before proceeding to the other eye in Step 3. The outcome is that the direct effects (represented by D) and the indirect effects (represented by I) are inline. There are two direct effects in the column for the right eye and two indirect effects in the column for the left eye up to the Snellen chart drill in Step 2.

Table 18.2 represents the arrangement of the direct and indirect effects after performing the Standard or Preliminary Drill. Suppose the wearing sequence also starts with the right eye. The patient performs the Distance Drill with the right eye in Step 1, the Distance Drill with the left eye in Step 2, and the Snellen Chart Drill with the right eye in Step 3. The outcome is that the direct and indirect effects are alternating. There are two direct effects and one indirect effect in the column for the right eye and two indirect effects and one direct effect in the column for the left eye up to the Snellen chart drill in Step 3.

In Table 18.1, there is no indirect effect on the right eye and no direct effect on the left eye after the right eye performs the Snellen chart drill for the first time in Step 2 (compared to the right eye performing the Snellen chart drill for the first time in Step 3 of Table 18.2). The absence of an indirect effect on the right eye prevents an overcorrection to the right crystalline lens, and the absence of a direct effect on the left eye prevents an overcorrection to the left crystalline lens. Although the prescription of the right eye is higher (since the patient starts with the weaker eye), the object of regard is 5 ft away.

18.3   RETRACTING THE ELONGATED EYE

There is a reduction in the direct effect's intensity by just having the right eye perform the Distance Drill in Step 1. The crystalline lens flattens out partially. There is still a gap between the focal point and the retina. It allows the Snellen Chart Drill in Step 2 to reduce more of the right eye's elongation.

The retraction of the left eye from a direct effect occurs in the same manner as the right eye. When the left eye performs the Snellen Chart Drill again in Step 4, the partial flattening of the lens in Step 3 allows for the eyeball's retraction. The crystalline lens flattened partially in Step 3 even though it received an indirect influence in Step 1. Unlike an alternating arrangement, the direct effect from the Distance Drill performed by the left eye in Step 3 did not follow immediately after the indirect effect from the Distance Drill performed by the right eye in Step 1. The indirect effect from the Distance Drill in Step 1 was interrupted when the right eye did the Snellen Chart Drill in Step 2. The indirect effect from the Snellen Chart Drill in Step 2 disconnected the indirect effect from the Distance Drill in Step 1. When the patient starts the Distance Drill over again in Step 3, it is incomplete. It only partially flattens the crystalline lens in the left eye.

18.4   REINFORCEMENT

The retraction of the right eyeball due to an indirect influence from the left eye in Step 4 reinforces the retraction from a direct influence on that eye in Step 2. The retraction of the left eyeball due to a direct influence in Step 4 reinforces the retraction from an indirect influence on that eye in Step 2. The indirect effect causes the left better eye to retract without having to influence the crystalline lens, and the indirect effect causes the right eye to retract without having to influence the crystalline lens. Implementing an indirect effect on the left better eye first tends to produce better results. Thus, the wearing sequence starts with the weaker eye.

18.5   APPLICATION OF THE DRILL

18.5.1   TREATING MILD MYOPIA

I would usually apply the Modified Preliminary Drill to treat a mild myopic eye of −0.50 D. The assumption is that the eyeball only deviated slightly. Instead of resorting to the Preliminary Drill prior to the Standard Drill to allow the participant to get used to the ortho C lenses, I would have him attempt the Modified Preliminary Drill instead. If the outcome of the Modified Preliminary Drill is not according to expectation, then it means the eyeball deviated a bit more. Then, I would have him try the Standard Drill. If it is according to expectations, then he would continue with the Modified Preliminary Drill. (Refer to the chapter *Case Examples* for more information.)

18.5.2   DIFFERENCES IN THE DRILL WHEN TREATING ANISOMETROPIA

The last two steps of the Modified Preliminary Drill to treat astigmatism are not included in the treatment for anisometropia. It is not necessary to look outside without any lenses on and perform the Distance Drill with each eye. The patient performs those steps when most of the deviation is in the crystalline lens. The last two steps readjust its flatness for distant focusing and compensation for astigmatism after performing the Snellen Chart Drill. Since the object of regard is 5 ft away, the lens tends to bulge slightly.

The time allotted for the Distance Drill in the treatment for anisometropia or anisometropia and astigmatism is 15 s versus 30 s in the treatment for myopia and astigmatism. The anisometropic eye is more sensitive to a flatter lens than the myopic eye. Remind the patient to complete the drill without interruption.

TABLE 18.1   Arrangement of Direct and Indirect Effects After Performing the Modified Preliminary Drill.

Drill's steps	Drill performed	Right eye	Left eye
1	Distance	D	I
2	Snellen	D	I
3	Distance	I	D
4	Snellen	I	D

TABLE 18.2 Arrangement of Direct and Indirect Effects After Performing the Preliminary Drill or Standard Drill.

Drill's steps	Drill performed	Right eye	Left eye
1	Distance	D	I
2	Distance	I	D
3	Snellen	D	I
4	Snellen	I	D

18.5.3 DIFFERENCE IN THE DRILL WHEN TREATING COMPOUND ANISOMETROPIA AND ANISOMETROPIC AMBLYOPIA

Another important difference in the Modified Preliminary Drill is when it is applied to treat compound anisometropia and anisometropic amblyopia, the wearing sequence is different. You would start with the better eye. It does not mean the weaker eye responds better to the drill. The neuropathway is different. (Refer to the chapter *Treating Anisometropia* for more information.)

18.6 THE MODIFIED PRELIMINARY DRILL TO TREAT SIMPLE ASTIGMATISM OR COMPOUND MYOPIA AND HIGH ASTIGMATISM

1. Wear the lens on the *weaker eye* only. Look outside at an object about 500 ft away. **Do not cover** the other eye that does not have the lens on. Keep both eyes open. Do the Distance Drill for 30 s.
2. With the lens still on the *weaker eye*, perform the Snellen Chart Drill. **Cover** the other eye. Hold the palm 2–3 in. from the eye. Keep both eyes open. Stand 5.0 ft away from the chart. Read line 7 five times at a rate of 1 s per letter. Then remove the lens.
3. Wear the lens on the *better eye* only. Look at an object about 500 ft away. **Do not cover** the other eye. Look at the same object in Step 1. Keep both eyes open. Do the Distance Drill for 30 s.
4. With the lens still on the *better eye*, perform the Snellen Chart Drill. **Cover** the other eye. Hold the palm 2–3 in. from the eye. Keep both eyes open. Stand 5.0 ft away from the chart. Read line 7 five times at a rate of 1 s per letter. Then remove the lens.

5. Without any lens on, look outside at an object about 500 ft away with the *weaker eye*. **Cover** the other eye. Look at the same object in Step 1. Leave a slight gap 2–3 in. from the eye. Keep both eyes open. Do the Distance Drill for 30 s.

6. Without any lens on, look outside at an object about 500 ft away with the *better eye*. **Cover** the other eye. Look at the same object in Step 1. Leave a slight gap 2–3 in. from the eye. Keep both eyes open. Do the Distance Drill for 30 s.

18.7   THE MODIFIED PRELIMINARY DRILL TO TREAT ANISOMETROPIA OR COMPOUND ANISOMETROPIA AND HIGH ASTIGMATISM

1. Wear the lens on the *weaker eye* only. Look outside at an object about 500 ft away. *Do not cover* the other eye that does not have the lens on. Keep both eyes open. Do the Distance Drill for 15 s.

2. With the lens still on the *weaker eye*, perform the Snellen Chart Drill. *Cover* the other eye. Hold the palm 2–3 in. from the eye. Keep both eyes open. Stand 5.0 ft away from the chart. Read line 7 five times at a rate of 1 s per letter. Then remove the lens.

3. Wear the lens on the *better eye* only. Look at an object about 500 ft away. *Do not cover* the other eye. Look at the same object in Step 1. Keep both eyes open. Do the Distance Drill for 15 s.

4. With the lens still on the *better eye*, perform the Snellen Chart Drill. *Cover* the other eye. Hold the palm 2–3 in. from the eye. Keep both eyes open. Stand 5.0 ft away from the chart. Read line 7 five times at a rate of 1 s per letter. Then remove the lens.

18.8   THE MODIFIED PRELIMINARY DRILL TO TREAT COMPOUND ANISOMETROPIA AND ANISOMETROPIC AMBLYOPIA

1. Wear the lens on the *better eye* only. Look outside at an object about 500 ft away. *Do not cover* the other eye that does not have the lens on. Keep both eyes open. Do the Distance Drill for 15 s.

2. With the lens still on the *better eye*, perform the Snellen Chart Drill. *Cover* the other eye. Hold the palm 2–3 in. from the eye.

Keep both eyes open. Stand 5.0 ft away from the chart. Read line 7 five times at a rate of 1 s per letter. Then remove the lens.

3. Wear the lens on the *weaker eye* only. Look at an object about 500 ft away. *Do not cover* the other eye. Look at the same object in Step 1. Keep both eyes open. Do the Distance Drill for 15 s.

4. With the lens still on the *weaker eye*, perform the Snellen Chart Drill. *Cover* the other eye. Hold the palm 2–3 in. from the eye. Keep both eyes open. Stand 5.0 ft away from the chart. Read line 7 five times at a rate of 1 s per letter. Then remove the lens.

KEYWORDS

- anisometropia
- simple astigmatism
- direct effect
- indirect effect
- inline
- alternating

CHAPTER 19

TREATING MILD AND MODERATE MYOPIA

ABSTRACT

The Standard Drill treats mild and moderate myopia from −0.75 D to −1.75 D. The prescription for each eye is the same. If there is a disparity between each eye, it is −0.25 D or less. The contact lens' flatness factor is equal to the absolute value of the prescription—or more specifically, to the absolute value of the sphere. The assumption is that patient's prescription is within the myopic model, and the deviation took place during postdevelopment. The conditions allows for the application of the multiplier effect.

In higher degrees of myopia, the tension of the oblique muscles increases. A flatter ortho C lens is required to loosen the oblique muscles sufficiently before you can effectively reverse the myopic shape of the eye. Such a lens poses a dilemma. A lens with a flatness of 3.75 D, for example, is outside the flatness tolerance. The meniscus is not adequate to allow a "focal point draw" before ortho K kicks in after the solution drains. (ortho C and ortho K do not mix.) The mild and moderate myopic eye does not have such a problem. The flatness factor is not that high. The highest is 1.75 D to treat the maximum range of moderate myopia.

19.1 THE FORMAT

Mild myopia is from −0.25 D to −0.75 D, and moderate myopia is from −1.00 D to −1.75 D. (Treatable mild myopia is from −0.50 D to −0.75 D.) Your patient's prescription gives a general idea of the problem. Mild myopia can be written as: Sphere: OD −0.50 D and OS −0.50 D, Cylinder: nil, Add: nil. In this example, the "sphere" does not reside mainly in one meridian as in the cylinder. Every meridian is off by −0.50 D in the right and left eye. If your patient informed you that her prescription is −0.50 D, she is actually saying that the sphere is −0.50 D. In the above example, there is no astigmatism (or "cylinder") or presbyopia (or "Add"). The acronym OD refers to your right eye and OS refers to your left eye. You would apply the Standard Drill to treat the problem.

19.2   FLATTENING THE CRYSTALLINE LENS' OCCLUDED NEUTRAL SHAPE

When one eye is covered, the lens takes on an occluded neutral shape in the open eye as well as the covered eye. Both lenses take on a rounder shape (Yee, 2011) . It accounts for why a myopee's visual acuity for each eye is slightly worse than the visual acuity for both eyes. Ortho C's ability to neurologically flatten the lens' occluded neutral shape is an important concept. There is more room for the lens to flatten, and that means it entices more of the eyeball in proportion to flatten.

When the "contact lens draw" initiated by the contact lens on the opened eye stimulates the ciliary muscle to relax in Step 1 of the Standard Drill, it is the lens' occluded neutral shape that flattens out. In turn, it also triggers the eyeball to reduce its elongation. The second myopic relationship also needs to reverse before the lens' occluded neutral shape remains flat. The phenomenon makes mild and moderate myopia easier to treat compared to myopia that mainly resides in the sclera or shared equally between the lens and sclera. It is easier to influence the smaller muscle that controls the lens (the ciliary muscle) than the larger muscles that control the eyeball (the oblique and rectus muscles).

The demonstration that the phenomenon takes place was given in the chapter *The Theory Behind the Standard Drill.* By treating the moderate myopic eye with just the first part of the Preliminary Drill, it only attends to the opened neutral shape of the crystalline lens. The flattening of the lens' open neutral shape does not necessarily flatten out the eyeball. The patient needs to cover one eye during the Standard Drill to expose the lens' occluded neutral shape—assuming the eye has a low resistance (to ortho C). If the lens has a high resistance, the lens's occluded neutral shape is the same as its open neutral shape.

19.3   THE TREATMENT

The following refractive errors are ranked according to the difficulty in treatment. Treating mild myopia actually starts with a prescription of −0.50 D. It is ironical that a prescription of −0.25 D is ranked at the end. It is the most difficult to treat, and I included its treatment for information only. I tend to apply the Modified Preliminary Drill to treat mild myopia of −0.50 D. The assumption is that the eyeball only deviated slightly. If the eyeball deviated slightly more, then the Standard Drill is the drill of choice. If the outcome of the Modified Preliminary Drill is not according to expectation, then you would try the Standard Drill.

The flatness factor depends on the prescription; the higher the prescription, the flatter the lens. The disparity in the prescription between the right and left eye also affects the flatness factor. The Standard Drill is effective if the disparity is up to −0.25 D. It is an indication that both eyes can be stimulated together in the first part of the drill. If the disparity is −0.50 D, it is an indication that it is a borderline case. The lens' flatness also depends on other refractive errors in addition to myopia—such as anisometropia and high astigmatism.

19.3.1   PSEUDOMYOPIA

Mild myopia is sometimes referred to as "pseudomyopia." When only the crystalline lenses had deviated, the tension of the oblique muscles can sometimes relax on its own without the assistance of a "contact lens draw." The excessive tension was not enough to alter the shape of the eyeball, and it may subside when the external adverse conditions are removed.

Perhaps the relationship between the lens and the eyeball formed a higher resistance against any change for the worse—such as during postdevelopment (when there is the tendency for the eyeball to shorten as the lens tends to bulge) as opposed to development (when there is the tendency for the lens to flatten out as the eyeball tends to bulge). Thus, the compensating factor of the eyeball during postdevelopment provides a higher resistance to the adverse form of myopia (which resides mainly in the eyeball). (Refer to the chapter *Treating Progressive Myopia* for more information on compensating factors and aggravating factors during postdevelopment and development.)

19.3.2   TREATING MILD MYOPIA –0.50 D

I would usually apply the Modified Preliminary Drill to treat a mild myopic eye of −0.50 D. The assumption is that the eyeball only deviated slightly. If the outcome is not according to expectation, then it means the eyeball deviated a bit more. Then I would have him try the Standard Drill. If it is according to expectations, then he would continue with the Modified Preliminary Drill. (Refer to the chapter *Case Examples* for more information.)

19.3.3   TREATING MILD AND MODERATE MYOPIA FROM –0.75 D TO –1.75 D

The Standard Drill is designed to treat myopia that falls into the −0.75 D to −1.75 D range. An ortho C lens' flatness for mild and moderate myopia is usually equal to the absolute value of the prescription. I qualified "usually" because there are exceptions. It depends on the disparity between the prescriptions for the right and left eye. If the prescription for each eye is the same or if the difference between them is −0.25 D, then the expected improvement in visual acuity and the retention period would be in the maximum range. The flatness factor is equal to the absolute value of the prescription for the right and left eye. For example, if the patient's prescription is OD −0.50 D and OS −0.75 D, the flatness for the right lens is 0.50 D and for the left lens is 0.75 D.

The duration for each step in the first part of the drill is 30 s. It ensures that the negative tear value does not have an adverse effect on the crystalline lens. (The artificial lighting also assists in the prevention.) The patient occludes each eye in the first and second part of the drill to expose the lens' occluded myopic shape. Monocular vision is more challenging than binocular vision in the myopic eye. It exposes the lens' occluded neutral shape to the multiplier effect.

The lenses are worn together in the first part of the drill to create a multiplier effect. The crystalline lens' occluded neutral shape needs to "shift" first before the eyeball "shifts." The "shift" in the eyeball in the first part of the drill reduces how much it needs to "shift" in the second part.

The second part of the Standard drill is equivalent to the second part of the Preliminary Drill. The lenses are worn one at a time. In the Standard

Drill, the better eye performs the Snellen Chart Drill first. In the Preliminary Drill and Modified Preliminary Drill, the weaker eye performs the drill first. Instruct the patient not to read line 7 too quickly in the second part of the drill (Steps 3 and 4). It is at a rate about 1.0 s per letter. It allows the number to come into focus before moving to the next number. Stand exactly 5.0 ft from the chart. It represents the degree of adjustment the eyeball needs to make. The eye converges slightly at that distance even though one eye is occluded; that is why both eyes are kept open. Tension is imparted to the rectus muscles during the convergence, and it assists in the retraction of the elongated eyeball.

In the last part of the drill, the crystalline lens is synchronized with the modified shape of the sclera when looking into the distance. The lens needs to be readjusted. It bulged slightly during the second part of the drill at 5.0 ft away from the object of regard to allow the sclera to become less elongated. The oblique muscles should still be sufficiently relaxed from the "contact lens draw" to allow the adjustment to take place before the tension settles. (Refer to the end of this chapter on how to perform the Standard Drill. Refer to the chapter *What to Do* on how to perform the supplementary drills that make up the Standard Drill: The Distance Drill and the Snellen Chart Drill.)

19.3.4 TREATING A DISPARITY OF –0.50 D BETWEEN THE RIGHT AND LEFT EYE

If the difference in the prescriptions between the right and left eye is -0.50 D, the disparity is outside the margin of error that allows the flatness factor to be equal to patient's prescription. The flatness factor for the better eye is equal to the absolute value of the prescription for that eye plus 0.25 D. The flatness factor for the weaker eye is equal to the absolute value of the prescription for that eye less 0.25 D. For example, if the prescription is OD -1.00 D and OS -1.50 D, the flatness for the right eye is 1.25 D and for the left eye is 1.25 D.

The imbalance between the right and left eye of -0.50 D does not qualify as anisometropia, but the disparity is just enough to justify applying the Modified Preliminary Drill. The patient can immediately perform the Modified Preliminary Drill without having to resort to the Preliminary Drill first. The Preliminary Drill may be a too intense. It can overcorrect the crystalline lens. A resistance can build up if you force the lens to flatten beyond how much it deviated.

19.3.5   TREATING A DISPARITY OF –0.75 D BETWEEN THE RIGHT AND LEFT EYE

If there is a disparity of −0.75 D between the right and left eye, you would treat the patient for anisometropia. Although the disparity does not qualify as anisometropia, you can still perform the treatment according to protocol. (Refer to the chapter *Treating Anisometropia*.)

19.3.6   TREATING MILD MYOPIA OF –0.25 D IN BOTH EYES

You have to be careful not to overcorrect the mild myopic shape of the lens or eyeball by exceeding the required flatness. You can only reinstate the neuromuscular message of the normal eye—not beyond normal. It is better to make it less flat than to make it too flat. If it is too flat, the negative effect is more noticeable with mild myopia.

I mentioned in the *Introduction* that you should pass up on attempting to treat a patient with a prescription of −0.25 D in both eyes. It would be even more difficult to deal with such a prescription if it resides in just one eye while the other eye is emmetropic. It is not feasible to design a lens for the emmetropic eye. The indirect influence of the lens on the weaker eye would overcorrect it.

The following procedure on how to treat it is for information only. It provides additional verification for ortho C. (Refer also to the chapter *Troubleshooting* for such a case example.)

It is more difficult to treat a prescription of OD −0.25 and OS −0.25 than the higher ranges of myopia since −0.25 D is closer to the emmetropic state. There is not much room for error.

One of the stipulations is that you can only correct the myopic eye within the range it deviated. As a demonstration, if you place a 0.50 flatter lens on an emmetropic eye, you are correcting something that does not need correction. Its visual acuity would deteriorate.

Although the prescription for each eye is the same, a difference in visual acuity can aggravate the problem. The weaker eye may see one line less on the Snellen chart (e.g., OD line 8 and OS line 7). To treat such as disparity, the flatness of the lens for the better eye would be on the steep

K, and the flatness of the lens for the weaker eye would be 0.25 D flatter than steep K. The right lens is on the steep K to prevent overcorrecting the crystalline lens. The steep K allows a wider margin of error compared to the mid K. If the patient sees equally well with each eye (e.g., OD line 7 and OS line 7), the lens' flatness for the right and left eye would be 0.25 D flatter than steep K.

The patient would perform just Steps 1 and 2 of the Standard Drill with the above lenses. Performing the other steps would overcorrect the eye. Remember to inform the patient to start with the better eye. When performing the First Resistance Test with the above lenses to verify the improvement in visual acuity, the patient would wear the lens in the weaker eye first. The wearing sequence changes when switching over to the Standard Drill. (Refer to the chapter *Troubleshooting* for such a case example.)

19.3.7   COMPOUND ASTIGMATISM AND MYOPIA

The "cylinder" portion of the prescription represents the amount of astigmatism. If the cylinder is −1.00 D or less and if the sphere is moderate, you would ignore it. The Standard Drill can partially correct it. The brain can compensate for the residual astigmatism. However, if the astigmatism is less than −1.00 D, it can still have an impact on mild myopia. With mild myopia of −0.75 D along with a cylinder of −0.50 D, for example, conduct the resistance tests to determine whether the patient should perform the Standard Drill or Modified Preliminary Drill. If there is no change in visual acuity after the First Resistance Test, it is a hint that the patient should perform the Modified Preliminary Drill. If the cylinder is −1.00 D or less with mild or moderate myopia, the lens' flatness factor is equal to the absolute value of the sphere. The thickness is 0.15 mm. If the cylinder is more than −1.00 D, refer to the *Specifications* for the range of flatness and to the chapter *Treating Astigmatism* on how to treat it.

19.3.8   COMPOUND PRESBYOPIA AND MYOPIA

If the patient has presbyopia on top of mild or moderate myopia, the amount of presbyopia is indicated in the "Add" portion of the prescription. If the Add is less than the sphere, you would ignore it. The flatness factor is equal to the absolute value of the sphere. The thickness is 0.15 mm. If the Add is more than the sphere, the main problem is presbyopia instead of mild myopia. The treatment is beyond the scope of this book and would be covered in a different publication.

19.3.9   TREATING A PARTIAL RESISTANCE

The treatment is optimum if the mild or moderate myopia is within the myopic model and has a low resistance. If the eye is slightly outside the myopic model, it may have a partial resistance to ortho C. The patient would perform a different drill under the following conditions:

- If a patient with a primary refractive error partially responds to the First Resistance Test by about one line and to the Second Resistance Test by about one line, then the recommended drill is the Modified Preliminary Drill.
- If a patient with a primary refractive error does not respond to the First Resistance Test, but there is a two or three-line improvement after the Second Resistance Test, then the recommended drill is the Modified Preliminary Drill.
- If a patient with a primary refractive error does not respond to the First, Second, or Third Resistance Test, but there is about a one-line improvement after the Fourth Resistance Test, then the recommended drill is the Modified Standard Drill.

The Modified Standard Drill is slightly different than the Standard Drill. The lenses are worn one at a time in the first part of the drill. The first part of the drill is similar to the Preliminary Drill. Thus, there is a reduction in intensity in Steps 1 and 2. The multiplier effect takes place in the second part of the drill instead of the first part. Both lenses are worn together in the second part of the drill. Thus, there is an increase in intensity in Steps 3 and 4. The assumption is that the eyeball deviated more than the lens.

19.4   THE DRILLS

The following are steps for the Standard Drill, Modified Preliminary Drill, and Modified Standard Drill.

19.4.1 THE STANDARD DRILL TO TREAT MILD AND MODERATE MYOPIA FROM –0.75 D TO –1.75 D

1. Wear both lenses. Look outside at an object about 500 or 1000 ft away with the *better eye*. (Look 500 ft away if you have moderate myopia. Look 1000 ft away if you have mild myopia) *Cover* the other eye. Hold the palm 2–3 in. from the eye to prevent instrument myopia. Keep both eyes open. Do the Distance Drill for 30 s.

2. With both lenses still on, look at an object about 500 or 1000 ft away with the *weaker eye*. *Cover* the other eye. Look at the same object in Step 1. Hold the palm 2–3 in. from the eye. Keep both eyes open. Do the Distance Drill for 30 s. Then take off the lens on the weaker eye.

3. With only the lens on the *better eye*, perform the Snellen Chart Drill. *Cover* the other eye. Hold the palm 2–3 in. from the eye. Keep both eyes open. Stand 5.0 ft away from the chart. Read line 7 five times at a rate of 1 s per letter. Then take the lens off.

4. Insert the lens on the *weaker eye* and perform the Snellen Chart Drill. *Cover* the other eye. Hold the palm 2–3 in. from the eye. Keep both eyes open. Stand 5.0 ft away from the chart. Read line 7 five times at a rate of 1 s per letter. Then take the lens off.

5. *Without* any lenses on, look outside at an object about 500 or 1000 ft away with *both* eyes. Look at the same object in Step 1. Do the Distance Drill for 1 min with both eyes. Not with each eye separately.

19.4.2 THE MODIFIED PRELIMINARY DRILL TO TREAT A DISPARITY IN PRESCRIPTION BETWEEN THE RIGHT AND LEFT EYE OF –0.50 D

1. Wear the lens on the *weaker eye* only. Look outside at an object about 500 ft away. **Do not cover** the other eye that does not have the lens on. Keep both eyes open. Do the Distance Drill for 30 s.

2. With the lens still on the *weaker eye*, perform the Snellen Chart Drill. **Cover** the other eye. Hold the palm 2–3 in. from the eye. Keep both eyes open. Stand 5.0 ft away from the chart. Read line 7 five times at a rate of 1 s per letter. Then remove the lens.

3. Wear the lens on the *better eye* only. Look at an object about 500 ft away. **Do not cover** the other eye. Look at the same object in Step 1. Keep both eyes open. Do the Distance Drill for 30 s.

4. With the lens still on the *better eye*, perform the Snellen Chart Drill. **Cover** the other eye. Hold the palm 2–3 in. from the eye. Keep both eyes open. Stand 5.0 ft away from the chart. Read line 7 five times at a rate of 1 s per letter. Then remove the lens.

5. Without any lens on, look outside at an object about 500 ft away with the *weaker eye*. **Cover** the other eye. Look at the same object in Step 1. Leave a slight gap 2–3 in. from the eye. Keep both eyes open. Do the Distance Drill for 30 s.

6. Without any lens on, look outside at an object about 500 ft away with the *better eye*. **Cover** the other eye. Look at the same object in Step 1. Leave a slight gap 2–3 in. from the eye. Keep both eyes open. Do the Distance Drill for 30 s.

19.4.3   THE MODIFIED STANDARD DRILL TO TREAT MILD AND MODERATE MYOPIA WITH A PARTIAL RESISTANCE THAT IS RESPONSIVE ONLY TO THE FOURTH RESISTANCE TEST

1. Wear the lens on the *weaker eye* only. Look outside at an object about 500 ft away. **Do not cover** the other eye. Keep both eyes open. Do the Distance Drill for 30 s. Then take the lens off.

2. Wear the lens on the *better eye* only. Look outside at an object about 500 ft away. **Do not cover** the other eye. Look at the same object in Step 1. Keep both eyes open. Do the Distance Drill for 30 s. Then insert the other lens back on.

3. With both lenses on, perform the Snellen Chart Drill with the *weaker eye*. **Cover** the other eye. Hold the palm 2–3 in. from the eye. Keep both eyes open. Stand 5.0 ft away from the chart. Read line 7 five times at a rate of 1 s per letter.

4. With both lenses on, perform the Snellen Chart Drill with the *better eye*. **Cover** the other eye. Hold the palm 2–3 in. from the eye. Keep both eyes open. Stand 5.0 ft away from the chart. Read line 7 five times at a rate of 1 s per letter. Take off the lenses.

5. Without any lenses on, look outside at an object about 500 ft away with *both* eyes. Look at the same object in Step 1. Do the Distance Drill for 1 min with both eyes. Not with each eye separately.

KEYWORDS

- **Standard Drill**
- **multiplier effect**
- **pseudomyopia**
- **mild myopia**
- **moderate myopia**
- **astigmatism**
- **presbyopia**

CHAPTER 20

TREATING ANISOMETROPIA

ABSTRACT

The Modified Preliminary Drill treats anisometropia, where the disparity between the right and left eye is −0.75 D or more. The drill also treats compound anisometropia and anisometropic amblyopia. The assumption is that patient's prescription is within the myopic model, and the deviation took place during postdevelopment. The conditions allow for the application of an inline direct and indirect effect.

Normally, the patient attempts the Preliminary Drill first. It prepares the eye for the Modified Preliminary Drill. The conventional definition for anisometropia is a difference of at least −1.00 D between the right and left eye. In reference to what can be treated by ortho C, a disparity of −0.75 also qualifies as anisometropia.

The treatable range is when one eye is moderate (from −1.00 D to −1.75 D) while the other eye is in the midrange (from −2.00 D to −2.75 D). In that range, the treatment is optimal when the better eye is −1.00 D or −1.25 D, and the weaker eye is −2.00 D or −2.25 D. It seems that the myopic range of the better eye determines the degree of correction for both eyes. Anisometropia is another exception where the flatness of the lens is not equal to the absolute value of the prescription.

20.1   THE EXTENT OF ANISOMETROPIA

Near-point stress not only induces nearsightedness, but it may also disassociate the eye from how it is supposed to function. Not only is there a severance in synchronization between the lens and sclera but also between the right and left eye. In some cases of anisometropia, there are features of amblyopia. There is something that prevents the eye from receiving the proper signal to bring an object into focus under certain conditions.

Apart from any deterioration to the nerves, there may be a link between instrument myopia and the ability of the eye to focus properly in the distance. I found that it affects the weaker eye with anisometropic amblyopia. If the patient covers the better eye completely, it can have a negative effect on the weaker eye. As the palm is held farther from the occluded eye, it improves the visual acuity of the open eye. The effect of instrument myopia becomes less and less as the palm of the hand is held farther and farther away. If the weaker eye was occluded, it usually does not have a negative influence on the visual acuity of the better eye. I was surprise to find that about half of my participants with anisometropia have traces of amblyopia. Perhaps anisometropia tends to progress to anisometropic amblyopia?

Some patients also have anisometropia and high astigmatism. Similar to treating moderate myopia and high astigmatism, there would be traces of residual myopia and astigmatism that become apparent in low lighting conditions. You may have to cut a pair of weaker glasses and have the patient adopt a technique called monovision in the interim. (Refer to the chapter *Treating Astigmatism* for more information.)

20.2   THE IMPACT OF NEAR-POINT STRESS ON THE WEAKER AND BETTER EYE

Although the weaker eye tends to become progressively worse when exposed to near-point stress, the better eye is not subjected to a similar rate of deterioration. Near-point stress indirectly impacts the better eye via the weaker eye. The increase in tension of the oblique muscles in the weaker eye spills over onto the better eye, but it does not alter its prescription right away. The better eye would still progress to a higher degree of myopia due to near-point stress, but it does not deteriorate as rapid as the weaker eye.

The visual acuity of a patient without anisometropia is different: the binocular visual acuity of a moderate myopic patient, for example, is better than the visual acuity of each eye by as much as one line on the Snellen chart even when the prescription for each eye is the same. Sometimes, the binocular visual acuity of an anisometropic patient is the opposite. The visual acuity of both eyes together tends to be lower than the visual acuity of the better eye. It is the prescription of the weaker eye that drags the binocular vision down. The binocular visual acuity, however, is higher than the visual acuity of the weaker eye.

20.3   THE CILIARY MUSCLE OF AN ANISOMETROPIC EYE

It seems that the tension of the ciliary muscle of the weaker eye is transmitted to the better eye. The excess tension of the ciliary muscle of the better eye did not cause the crystalline lens to deviate as much as the weaker eye—even though the ciliary muscle of the better eye is as thick as the weaker eye. The bulged shape of the crystalline lens is not in proportion to the tension of the ciliary muscle. Kuchem et al. (2013) found that the better eye has the same ciliary muscle thickness as the higher myopic eye with a longer axial length. The subjects were between 18 and 40 years.

If the tension of the ciliary muscle is high in the better eye, the tension of the oblique muscles should also be high in the attempt to relieve that tension; but the increase in tension of the ciliary muscle was not initiated by the crystalline lens. It was indirectly induced by the other eye. It poses a dilemma. A lens with a flatness factor designed according to the weaker eye to relax the ciliary muscle may have a negative impact on the crystalline lens in the better eye due to the negative tear factor (from a lens that is too flat). Designing a lens that is less flat may not adequately relax the ciliary muscle.

20.4   THE TREATMENT

20.4.1   ANISOMETROPIA

The first problem you need to resolve is the tension of the ciliary muscle of both eyes. Their thickness is the same. The myopic shape of the crystalline lens and eyeball of the better eye, however, is not in proportion to the thickness of the ciliary muscle. It was induced by the weaker eye. The Preliminary Drill is usually performed first to relax the ciliary muscle of both eyes and flatten the crystalline lens of the better eye to ensure that it can take a flatter lens. The patient performs the Modified Preliminary Drill after performing the Preliminary Drill twice a week for about 2 weeks.

20.4.1.1   A DISPARITY OF −1.00 D

Anisometropia is a disparity in prescription between the right and left eye of −1.00 D or more. The treatment is optimal when the better eye is −1.00

D or −1.25 D, and the weaker eye is −2.00 D or −2.25 D. If one eye is −1.00 D and the other eye is −2.00 D, for example, the client would often experience about a three-line improvement in binocular visual acuity after performing the Modified Preliminary Drill. The flatness factor for both lenses is equal to the absolute value of the weaker eye. In the above example, the flatness factor for the right and left eye is still 2.00 D. It is the maximum flatness. If the patient's prescription is OD −1.50 D and OS −2.25 D, for example, the flatness factor for the right and left eye is still 2.00 D regardless of the prescription of the weaker eye (within the midrange from −2.00 D to −2.75 D). Do not go beyond 2.00 D. A further qualification to ensure that the negative tear value does not have a negative impact on the better eye is that the myopic range of the better eye should start at −0.50 D.

20.4.1.2   A DISPARITY OF −0.75 D

If there is a disparity of −0.75 D between the right and left eye, you would treat the patient for anisometropia. Although the disparity does not fall under the conventional definition for anisometropia, you can still perform the treatment according to protocol. The patient would perform the Preliminary Drill first for 2 weeks (for two times a week) before proceeding to the Modified Preliminary Drill.

20.4.1.3   DISPARITY OF −0.50 D

Although a disparity of −0.50 D between the right and left eye does not qualify as anisometropia, it can still be treated by the Modified Preliminary Drill. The patient would immediately adopt the Modified Preliminary Drill. It is not necessary to perform the Preliminary Drill first. (Refer to the chapter *Treating Mild and Moderate Myopia* for more information.)

20.4.1.4   ONE EYE IS MODERATE AND THE OTHER EYE IS IN THE MIDRANGE

If one eye's prescription is moderate and the other eye is in the midrange and the disparity between them is at least −0.75 D, the treatment is more effective than treating anisometropia in the higher ranges. It is ironic that it is also sometimes more effective than treating anisometropia in the lower ranges.

20.4.1.5   ONE EYE IS MILD OR MODERATE AND THE OTHER EYE IS MODERATE

If the prescription of one eye is mild or moderate and the other eye is in the moderate range with a disparity of at least −0.75 D, the flatness factor for both lenses takes on the absolute value of the prescription of the weaker eye. For example, if the right eye is −0.50 D and the other eye is −1.50 D, then the flatness factor for the right and left lens is 1.50 D. You would still treat the patient for anisometropia. The success of the treatment depends on the prescription of the weaker eye. The higher negative tear factor impacts the mild myopic eye more than the moderate myopic eye.

20.4.1.6   ONE EYE IS −0.25 D AND THE OTHER EYE IS MODERATE

Care should be taken when the better eye is −0.25 D and the other eye is in the moderate range with a disparity of at least −0.75 D. I suggest that you pass up treating such a prescription. If the weaker left eye's prescription is −1.25 D, placing a lens with a flatness of 1.25 D on the better eye may overcorrect that eye. Although an anisometropic eye is different, the margin of error is less.

If the indirect influence from the lens on the weaker eye was not sufficient to activate the ciliary muscle of the better eye by relaxing the oblique muscles, then a flatter ortho C lens worn on the better eye can cause the crystalline lens to deteriorate. The negative tear layer from the lens on the better eye is comparable to wearing a −1.25 D lens. The binocular visual acuity would be affected since it is a function of the visual acuity of the better right eye.

You may never come across a prescription of OD −0.25 D and OS −1.25 D. In all the years, I spent researching the treatment for anisometropia, I only saw it once. It changed to OD −1.25 D and OS −2.25 D by the time he decided to try the procedure months later. Anisometropia progresses rapidly; by the time the patient notices it, the prescription would have progressed to a higher range.

20.4.2   COMPOUND ANISOMETROPIA AND ANISOMETROPIC AMBLYOPIA

In the treatment for severe myopia, I have the option of increasing the intensity of the drill by increasing the lens' flatness factor. There is the temptation to do the same when treating anisometropia plus anisometropic amblyopia when the Preliminary Drill becomes ineffective after a few weeks, but do not. You should actually be switching to a less intense drill once a resistance builds up: the Modified Preliminary Drill. It produces better results. Besides, it is difficult to assign a flatness factor to treat anisometropic amblyopia. You would not know the extent of the amblyopia. Unlike strabismic amblyopia, the eye appears normal. It is difficult to measure the amount of deviation. (Refer to *Troubleshooting* for more information.)

Similar to anisometropia, the client with anisometropia and anisometropic amblyopia would often experience a three-line improvement in visual acuity binocularly after applying the Modified Preliminary Drill. Sometimes, it would become sharper than a patient with just anisometropia. It is ironic that a patient with anisometropia and anisometropic amblyopia would benefit more from ortho C. It seems that it is more neurologically entrenched; by resetting the correct neurological message, the patient tends to benefit more.

20.4.2.1   REVERSE THE WEARING SEQUENCE

The proper wearing sequence would apply during the Preliminary Drill; but when switching over to the Modified Preliminary Drill to treat anisometropia plus anisometropic amblyopia while keeping the same wearing sequence, the patient would see better with the weaker eye after the drill. It is an indication to switch the wearing sequence. He would wear the lens in the better eye first and then finish with the lens in the weaker eye instead. It is not because the weaker eye is more receptive to ortho C than the better eye. The neuropathway is different. (Refer to the chapter Troubleshooting for more information.) Once the patient starts the first part of the drill with the better eye and completes the second part of the drill with the weaker eye, the visual acuity would further improve and become proportionate. He would still see slightly better with the better eye, but the disparity is less. Often the binocular vision would be much sharper than an anisometropic eye. The patient with compound anisometropia and anisometropic amblyopia would often find that driving during the evening without glasses is much clearer and last much longer (usually just a bit over 2 weeks) than a patient with just anisometropia.

20.5   THE DRILLS

The following are the steps for the Preliminary Drill and Modified Preliminary Drill to treat anisometropia. The steps for the Modified Preliminary Drill are also included to treat compound anisometropia and anisometropic amblyopia. The wearing sequence is different from treating anisometropia without anisometropic amblyopia.

20.5.1   THE PRELIMINARY DRILL TO TREAT ANISOMETROPIA

1. Wear the lens on the *weaker eye* only. Look outside at an object about 500 ft away. **Do not cover** the other eye. Keep both eyes open. Do the Distance Drill for 15 s. Then take the lens off.
2. Wear the lens on the *better eye* only. Look outside at an object about 500 ft away. **Do not cover** the other eye. Look at the same object in Step 1. Keep both eyes open. Do the Distance Drill for 15 s. Then take the lens off.
3. Wear the lens on the *weaker eye* only. Perform the Snellen Chart Drill with the *weaker eye* first. **Cover** the other eye. Hold the palm about 2–3 in. from the eye. Keep both eyes open. Stand 5.0 ft away from the chart. Read line 7 five times at a rate of 1 s per letter. Then take the lens off.
4. Wear the lens on the *better eye* only. Perform the Snellen Chart Drill with the *better eye*. **Cover** the other eye. Hold the palm about 2–3 in. from the eye. Keep both eyes open. Stand 5.0 ft away from the chart. Read line 7 five times at a rate of 1 s per letter. Then take the lens off.
5. Without any lens on, look outside at an object about 500 ft away with the *weaker eye*. **Cover** the other eye. Look at the same object in Step 1. Leave a slight gap 2–3 in. from the eye. Keep both eyes open. Do the Distance Drill for 30 s.
6. Without any lens on, look outside at an object about 500 ft away with the *better eye*. **Cover** the other eye. Look at the same object

in Step 1. Leave a slight gap 2–3 in. from the eye. Keep both eyes open. Do the Distance Drill for 30 s.

20.5.2 THE MODIFIED PRELIMINARY DRILL TO TREAT ANISOMETROPIA

1. Wear the lens on the *weaker eye* only. Look outside at an object about 500 ft away. **Do not cover** the other eye that does not have the lens on. Keep both eyes open. Do the Distance Drill for 15 s.
2. With the lens still on the *weaker eye*, perform the Snellen Chart Drill. **Cover** the other eye. Hold the palm 2–3 in. from the eye. Keep both eyes open. Stand 5 ft away from the chart. Read line 7 five times at a rate of 1 s per letter. Then remove the lens.
3. Wear the lens on the *better eye* only. Look at an object about 500 ft away. **Do not cover** the other eye. Look at the same object in Step 1. Keep both eyes open. Do the Distance Drill for 15 s.
4. With the lens still on the *better eye*, perform the Snellen Chart Drill. **Cover** the other eye. Hold the palm 2–3 in. from the eye. Keep both eyes open. Stand 5 ft away from the chart. Read line 7 five times at a rate of 1 s per letter. Then remove the lens.

20.5.3 THE MODIFIED PRELIMINARY DRILL TO TREAT COMPOUND ANISOMETROPIA AND ANISOMETROPIC AMBLYOPIA

1. Wear the lens on the *better eye* only. Look outside at an object about 500 ft away. *Do not cover* the other eye that does not have the lens on. Keep both eyes open. Do the Distance Drill for 15 s.
2. With the lens still on the *better eye*, perform the Snellen Chart Drill. *Cover* the other eye. Hold the palm 2–3 in. from the eye. Keep both eyes open. Stand 5.0 ft away from the chart. Read line 7 five times at a rate of 1 s per letter. Then remove the lens.
3. Wear the lens on the *weaker eye* only. Look at an object about 500 ft away. *Do not cover* the other eye. Look at the same object in Step 1. Keep both eyes open. Do the Distance Drill for 15 s.
4. With the lens still on the *weaker eye*, perform the Snellen Chart Drill. *Cover* the other eye. Hold the palm 2–3 in. from the eye.

Keep both eyes open. Stand 5.0 ft away from the chart. Read line 7 five times at a rate of 1 s per letter. Then remove the lens.

KEYWORDS

- **Modified Preliminary Drill**
- **anisometropia**
- **anisometropic amblyopia**
- **disparity**
- **near-point stress**
- **ciliary muscle**
- **monovision**

CHAPTER 21

TREATING ASTIGMATISM

ABSTRACT

The Modified Preliminary Drill also treats simple astigmatism, compound myopia and high astigmatism, and compound anisometropia and high astigmatism. The assumption is that the patient's prescription is within the myopic model. The contact lens' flatness factor to treat "compound astigmatism" is equal to the absolute value of the "sphere" if the astigmatism is low. If the astigmatism is high, the flatness factor is equal to the absolute value of the "sphere" plus a compensating value—usually 0.25 D. (Refer to the chapter *Specifications*.)

21.1   HOW IT CAME ABOUT

No one knows the cause of astigmatism because it is hidden in the cause for myopia. Near-point stress can also contribute to astigmatism. The second myopic relationship entices the rectus muscles to relax to allow the eyeball to elongate (to alleviate the tension of the ciliary muscle during close-up work). Sometimes the tension of the rectus muscles does not "loosen" uniformly. The horizontal rectus muscles often do not offer enough slack compared to the vertical rectus muscles. The misalignment may induce astigmatism along with myopia.

The culprit is likely the vertical rectus muscles, and it contributes to astigmatism when the relaxation of those muscles results in a steeper cornea along that meridian. The horizontal rectus muscles maintained their tension and entice the cornea along that meridian to retain their original shape. One of the horizontal muscles, the lateral rectus, is innervated by the sixth cranial nerve (or C6) instead of the third cranial nerve (or C3) which is common with all the other rectus muscles. It may explain why it does not offer enough slack to comply with the rest of the rectus muscles.

The horizontal pair of rectus muscles as a whole remains relatively taut regardless if the medial rectus, the other horizontal muscle, offers some slack (since it is innervated by C3). The cornea tends to uphold its spherical shape along the horizontal meridian (Yee, 2012).

In most cases, astigmatism is mainly due to the distortion of the cornea, and it is referred to as "corneal astigmatism." In some cases, it is mainly due to the distortion of the crystalline lens, and it is termed "lenticular astigmatism." Astigmatism can exist by itself, or it can be combined with myopia or hyperopia. The former is called "simple astigmatism," and the latter is called "compound astigmatism." Simple astigmatism is further broken down into "simple myopic astigmatism" and "simple hyperopic astigmatism."

Unlike an eye with a primary refractive error, the crystalline lens of a compound astigmatic eye may not inherit most of the myopia. Instead, it may have inherited some modification while attempting to compensate for corneal astigmatism. Ortho C attempts to take advantage of the lens' natural tendency to compensate for the astigmatism by amplifying the compensation (Yee, 2012).

21.2   CORNEAL ASTIGMATISM

With corneal astigmatism, the distortion of a distant image is mainly due to the cornea. The misalignment in the tension of the rectus muscles physically spreads onto the cornea to induce corneal astigmatism. The vertical curvature of the cornea is steep. It bulges more due to the looseness of the vertical pair of rectus muscles. The horizontal curvature is flat since the horizontal rectus muscles are still relatively taut.

Neurologically, the misalignment in the tension of the rectus muscles is passed onto the crystalline lens. Since the ciliary muscle and the rectus muscles are innervated by the common cranial nerve C3, the brain modifies the curvature of the crystalline lens to partially compensate for the uneven cornea. The crystalline lens can naturally offset astigmatism up to around −1.00 D (Yee, 2012). There are experiments where the emmetropic eyes can adjust to astigmatic goggles placed over them for about 10 min. After removal, there is another adjustment period to regain emmetropia. But do not attempt the experiment. You are actually inducing lenticular astigmatism, and it may become permanent.

For corneal astigmatism over −1.00 D, ortho C takes advantage of the motor cortex's ability to compensate for some of the astigmatism. A "contact lens draw" attempts to amplify this compensation by stimulating the ciliary muscle to further "flatten" the crystalline lens along a certain meridian to neutralize the astigmatism (Yee, 2012). When the "draw" "loosens" the oblique muscles, the brain reinterprets the eye to be in distant mode. If the eye was myopic, it would attempt to "flatten" the crystalline lens uniformly; but if it was astigmatic, it would attempt to adjust the crystalline lens along a specific meridian to offset the steepest meridian on the cornea.

21.3   LENTICULAR ASTIGMATISM

With lenticular astigmatism, the distortion of a distant image is mainly due to the crystalline lens instead of the cornea. Similar to corneal astigmatism, the misalignment in tension of the rectus muscles spills over onto the cornea. The distortion, however, is different from corneal astigmatism. The horizontal meridian is steeper and the vertical meridian is flatter.

The horizontal rectus muscles are looser than the vertical rectus muscles in compliance to the tension of the oblique muscles of the myopic eye. The cornea's horizontal curvature would be steep, and the vertical curvature would be flat. The tension of the horizontal rectus muscles complied with the increase in tension of the oblique muscles. It is unusual for the horizontal rectus muscles to offer that much slack. Usually, the vertical rectus muscles are looser than the horizontal rectus muscles as in the case of corneal astigmatism.

Unlike corneal astigmatism, the difficulty in attempting to naturally compensate for the horizontal meridian of the cornea is probably due to the difference in innervation of the two horizontal rectus muscles. The horizontal rectus muscles are made up of the medial rectus and lateral rectus. The lateral rectus muscle is innervated by the sixth cranial nerve (or C6) instead of C3 which is common with all the other rectus muscles and the ciliary muscle.

The lateral rectus attempts to flatten the cornea by maintaining its tension while the medial rectus encourages the cornea to bulge by giving up some of its tension. When the latter predominates, the outcome is a steeper cornea along that meridian. The horizontal rectus muscles offer more slack overall compared to the other pair of vertical rectus muscles. In response to the horizontal steepness of the cornea, C3 attempts to entice the crystalline lens to become thinner horizontally along that meridian. The ciliary muscle does not act independently when it attempts to compensate for the corneal astigmatism. The rectus muscles map out the specific meridian where the adjustment needs to be made on the lens.

If the deviation is along the horizontal axis of the cornea or close to it, the crystalline lens cannot compensate for the steepness due to the difference in innervation between the two horizontal rectus muscles. As a result, the lens bulged instead of flatten for distance focusing (perhaps due to an excessive "effort to see"). It aggravates the astigmatism instead of compensating for it. The outcome is lenticular astigmatism (Yee, 2013a).

The procedure for treating lenticular astigmatism is the same as the procedure for treating corneal astigmatism. In the case of lenticular astigmatism, the intention is not to compensate for the astigmatism. The lens cannot naturally compensate for the distortion of the cornea if the deviation is due to the steepness along the horizontal axis or along a meridian close to it. Ortho C would have to correct the crystalline lens along that meridian independent of the cornea (Yee, 2013a). Again, with simple astigmatism, you do not have to alter the sclera since it did not assume a myopic shape; but similar to treating cases of mild myopia, you may have to reinforce its shape. Thus you have to assign a drill which is not as intense as the Standard Drill.

21.4   SIMPLE ASTIGMATISM

Simple astigmatism exists by itself. The two focal points from a distant image are projected by the difference in curvatures along two major meridians on the anterior surface of the cornea. One of them is the steepest (to comply with the tendency to become myopic) and the other is the flattest (to comply with the tendency to remain emmetropic). The former's focal point is in front of the retina, and the latter's focal point is on the retina. The distortion in vision is due to the disparity created by two focal points. The one that is in front of the retina also causes an object to be blur.

Simple astigmatism can be written as PL -1.00×180. In this example, there is no sphere. It is PL (or "plano"). The cylinder is -1.00 D in the $180°$

meridian. The flatter part of the cornea is along the 180° axis. You would probably never come across such a prescription if you do not fit eyeglasses or contact lenses regularly. It tends to progress to compound astigmatism before it starts to bother the patient enough to have it checked.

21.5 COMPOUND ASTIGMATISM

Compound astigmatism is a combination of astigmatism and myopia or hyperopia. Suppose your client has moderate myopia, and the astigmatism is −1.00 D or less. Do not adjust the base curve of the lens to account for the astigmatism. Just treat the problem as moderate myopia. If the astigmatism is over −1.00 D, you have to take it into account in addition to the sphere. You have to adjust for the astigmatism by designing the lens a bit flatter. The drill is still the same. (Refer to the chapter *Specifications* for the flatness factor for the specific compound astigmatism.)

If the patient has high presbyopia and high lenticular astigmatism on top of mild or moderate myopia, ortho C may induce double vision. There are too many negative variables: lenticular astigmatism and high presbyopia as well as myopia. All of those variables affect the crystalline lens. What may induce the double vision is the lenticular astigmatism. Such a prescription can be written as −1.25 − 1.50 × 90 with +2.00 addition (ADD). The presence of lenticular astigmatism is hinted at by the 90° axis written in the prescription. Even if the ADD is less than the sphere, I still suggest you do not treat this type of compound astigmatism.

21.6 REDUCE THE EFFORT OF COMPENSATION

Ortho C tends to physically align the misalignment in the tension of the rectus muscles, but any reduction in the difference in tension may not be immediately reflected on the cornea. Over time, however, the "flexing" of the rectus muscles with the ortho C lens on and the "letting go" after removal can increase the tensile strength of the pair of rectus muscles in reference to the cornea's steepest meridian. There may be a sufficient reduction in the misalignment in tension of the rectus muscles to physically reduce the difference in the distortion of the cornea. Although it is usually a partial reduction, it is enough to lower the effort imposed on the ciliary muscle to compensate for the corneal astigmatism. It also makes it easier to maintain the correction for lenticular astigmatism.

21.7   THE TREATMENT

21.7.1   TREATING SIMPLE ASTIGMATISM

To treat simple astigmatism, the lens' flatness factor is equal to the absolute value of the "cylinder" prescription. For example, if the prescription for the right eye is PL −0.50 × 180 and for the left eye is PL −0.75 × 180, the flatness factor for the right lens is 0.50 D and the left lens is 0.75 D. The astigmatism in each eye can be the same or different. If the astigmatism for each eye is the same, conduct a Visual Acuity Test to determine the wearing schedule. One eye is likely to see clearer compared to the other—even if it is just half a line clearer. The patient would wear the lens for the weaker eye first.

The patient would perform the Modified Preliminary Drill. The patient does not have to alter the sclera It did not assume a myopic shape. Similar to treating mild myopia, the drill adjusts the eyeball slightly to reinforce its spherical shape. The motor cortex is also able to distinguish whether the treatment is for corneal astigmatism or lenticular astigmatism. You do not have to do anything different.

21.7.2   TREATING COMPOUND MYOPIA AND LOW ASTIGMATISM

The patient can usually perform the Standard Drill for astigmatism up to −0.50 D in an eye with moderate myopia. By being able to perform the Standard Drill, it is an indication that the brain can compensate for the astigmatism. It also means that the disparity in prescription between the right and left eye is less than −0.50 D.

If the sphere is −1.25 D and the astigmatism is −0.50 D, the "compound astigmatism" can be written as −1.25 − 0.50 180. The axis at 180° suggests the presence of corneal astigmatism. The flatness factor in this example is equal to the absolute value of the sphere or 1.25 D according to the chapter *Specifications*. I am often asked how the so-called one-third rule fits into the picture. According to the literature, if the astigmatism is more than one-third of the sphere, then the patient may experience distortion when attempting to bring a distant object into focus by just correcting the sphere—if I just correct for −1.25 D in the above example and not for the −0.50 D cylinder. I found that it applies to wearing a conventional soft contact lens and not to ortho C.

The compensation here is different from the compensation mentioned in the discussion on corneal astigmatism. Corneal astigmatism is the difference between the horizontal and vertical curvature on the K reading. When the astigmatism shows up on the prescription, as in the above example, it is the residual astigmatism after the brain tried its best to compensate for the corneal astigmatism. The corneal astigmatism is probably over −1.00 D. What is left over after compensation is −0.50 D of cylinder. We are asking ortho C to increase the compensation.

A borderline case may exist when the sphere is −1.00 D and the cylinder is −0.50 D. You need to perform a resistance test to determine which drill is more effective—the Standard Drill or the Modified Preliminary Drill. After performing the First Resistance Test, check the patient's visual acuity. The lack of any change in visual acuity is an indication that astigmatism interfered with the test. It also indicates that it will likely interfere with the Standard Drill. The First Resistance Test is actually the first part of the Preliminary Drill, and the first part of the Preliminary Drill is compatible with the Standard Drill. If it does not register an improvement or if the improvement does not last for more than a few minutes, the Modified Preliminary Drill is more appropriate than the Standard Drill.

21.7.3   TREATING COMPOUND MYOPIA AND HIGH ASTIGMATISM

There is an exception to what I said about being able to neurologically compensate for astigmatism up to −0.50 D. When the sphere is mild (−0.50 D or −0.75 D) and the astigmatism is equal or almost equal to it, apply the Modified Preliminary Drill. The cylinder may interfere with the Standard Drill even though it is less than −1.00 D. A mild myopic eye is more sensitive to astigmatism. The visual cortex considers the cylinder as high even though it is −0.50 D because it is over 50% of the sphere. The lens' flatness is equal to the flatness factor of the sphere. You do not have to account for the cylinder. If the prescription was $-0.75 - 0.50 \times 180$, the lens' flatness would be equal to the absolute value of the sphere (or 0.75 D). (Refer to the chapter *Specifications*.)

If the astigmatism is more than -1.00 D in the mild or moderate myopic eye, the lens' flatness is more than the flatness factor of the sphere. The patient would perform the Modified Preliminary Drill. If the prescription was $-1.25 - 1.50 \times 180$, the lens' flatness would be more than the absolute value of the sphere. According to the chapter *Specifications*, the flatness factor is equal to the absolute value of the sphere plus 0.25 D (which is equal to 1.50 D).

Although you are treating both the astigmatism and the myopia, there may be some residual myopia afterwards. The drill attends mainly to the astigmatism. Unlike the Standard Drill, the Modified Preliminary Drill does not start to reduce the elongated eyeball until the patient applies the Snellen chart drill. In the upper moderate myopic range such as -1.50 D or -1.75 D with a cylinder over -1.00 D, you may have to give the patient a pair of weaker glasses (usually -0.50 D or -0.75 D) for the blackboard, projected diagrams in artificial light, and for nighttime activities.

21.7.4   TREATING ANISOMETROPIA AND HIGH ASTIGMATISM

When high astigmatism is mixed in with anisometropia, the Preliminary Drill is usually not that effective. It mainly attends to anisometropia but not astigmatism. You would have to resort to the Modified Preliminary Drill. It treats anisometropia as well as high astigmatism. I also had success treating a combination of anisometropia, anisometropic amblyopia, and high astigmatism with the Modified Preliminary Drill. By the third application, an autorefractor would indicate that there is a significant improvement in the sphere, but the cylinder may remain the same since the lens was bypassed. In a subjective exam such as a visual acuity test, it would indicate that the crystalline lens would mask the astigmatism.

Consider the following prescription for the right and left eye: OD $-1.00 - 1.50 \times 180$ and OS $-2.00 - 0.50 \times 180$. The flatness factor is equivalent to the absolute value of the sphere of the weaker eye which is 2.00 D. The eye is in the midrange, and the flatness factor is the maximum. There is a disparity of -1.00 D in the cylinder (which is the measurement for the astigmatism) as well as in the sphere (the measurement for the myopia). The wearing sequence is the left eye first and then the right. The weaker eye is the eye with the higher sphere which is the left eye. Even if the cylinder is higher on the right eye, you would still go by the higher sphere. He sees worse out of that eye. Although the wearing sequence changes in an eye with anisometropia and anisometropic amblyopia, it defaults to the normal wearing sequence when the astigmatism is the predominant factor.

There may still be a difference in prescription between the right and left eye after the first few applications, but that is okay. The disparity in the short term is due to the better eye improving at a quicker rate. Also the drill attends to the cylinder more than the myopia. The weaker eye tends to lag behind. Its myopia is higher. As with treating myopia and high astigmatism, the eye may have residual myopia.

The patient adapts to the disparity by inheriting a technique called monovision. It is usually proposed to clients who cannot see objects close-up. An eye care specialist would fit the dominant eye with a contact lens to see far away. Close objects are blurrier for that eye. He would then fit the other eye with a contact lens to see objects close-up. Distant objects are blurrier for that eye. It appears that the patient is focusing with one eye but that is not the case. He adapts to both the distance and near.

After applying the Modified Preliminary Drill, the patient also sees well in the distance and close-up equally well with his binocular vision. It overrides what he can and cannot see with his monocular vision. The difference with an anisometropic eye and a presbyopic eye as in the above example is that prior to the treatment, one of the anisometropic eye sees better than the other whereas both presbyopic eye were equally out of focus. Thus the anisometropic patient had already adapted to monovision.

21.7.5   IT STIMULATES THE CRYSTALLINE LENS AND EYEBALL DIFFERENTLY

The Modified Preliminary Drill stimulates the ciliary muscle differently compared to the other drills. The first part of the Standard Drill is too intense. The mild and moderate myopic eye with a high cylinder does not require a multiplier effect to reverse how much it deviated. It is not necessary to expose the occluded myopic shape of the lens by covering the other eye. The Modified Preliminary Drill deals with the lens' astigmatic shape via its open neutral shape. The Preliminary Drill also stimulates the lens' open neutral shape, but the alternating sequence of the direct and indirect influences are too intense.

In Table 18.1 (in the chapter *The Theory Behind the Modified Preliminary Drill*), the Distance Drill is incomplete when the Snellen Chart Drill is implemented for the first time in Step 2. The Distance Drill was only performed on the right eye—assuming the wearing sequence starts with the right eye. The direct effect on that eye in Step 1 maps out the proper axis where the adjustment is to be made on the crystalline lens (Yee, 2012). If there was also an indirect effect from the other eye after Step 1, it would interrupt which meridian to flatten out. In order for the right lens to compensate for the astigmatism, only the direct effect is required. An alternating influence completes the Distance Drill and Snellen Chart Drill as in Table 18.2. It is better suited for myopia that has little or no astigmatism on the right or left eye.

The direct effect also map out the axis to treat the misalignment of the rectus muscles in Step 2 via the Snellen chart drill (Yee, 2012). The retraction of the eyeball can only be implemented when one pair of rectus muscles exert more of an influence than the other pair. When the eyeball elongated, one pair of rectus muscles relaxed more than the other pair. It is that pair that has to exert more tension than the other pair. The eyeball does not begin to retract until Step 2. In Step 1, only the lens' open neutral shape was activated when both eyes were looking at an object in the distance. In Step 2, the lens takes on an occluded neutral shape when the patient covers the other eye.

The drill tends to undercorrect the myopia. It deals with it only when it attempts to realign the rectus muscles to retract the eyeball. In high compound astigmatism such as a sphere of −1.50 D or −1.75 D and a high cylinder such as −1.25 D or more, the patient may need a pair of weaker glasses in the −0.50 D or −0.75 D range for settings that simulate night time conditions such as the blackboard in a classroom lit only by artificial light, a projected diagram in a dim room, et cetera. There may be residual myopia in the lens and eyeball not attended to effectively by the Modified Preliminary Drill.

21.7.6   VERIFICATION

I relied on a pretest posttest design in the chapter *Case Examples* to provide verification as well as well as a sample guide. Instead of a visual acuity test, you can also conduct a test with an autorefractor before the patient performs the drill. An autorefraction is an objective measurement where the patient does not give any input. It eliminates bias (from both the patient and the examiner). It only takes a few minutes to measure. It bypasses the crystalline lens by having it assume a neutral shape. Thus, the measurement essentially represents the axial length of the eyeball.

After performing the drill a few times, take another autorefractor reading. You would find that the myopia, or the "sphere", is much lower. Similar to myopia and high astigmatism, a reduction in the cylinder would show up only if the distortion is high. If the distortion is low (but regarded as high in relation to the sphere), it tends to remain unchanged. The crystalline lens can compensate for it, but it would not show up in the measurements when the lens is in a neutral shape. The compensation takes place only when there is a "focal point draw." (Refer to the chapter *Troubleshooting* for an application of the Modified Preliminary Drill in the treatment of high astigmatism induced by TBI.)

21.8   THE DRILLS

The following are the steps for the Standard Drill to treat compound astigmatism with a low cylinder and the steps for the Modified Preliminary Drill to treat simple astigmatism and compound astigmatism with a high cylinder.

21.8.1   THE STANDARD DRILL TO TREAT COMPOUND MYOPIA AND ASTIGMATISM WITH A LOW CYLINDER

1. Wear both lenses. Look outside at an object about 500 or 1000 ft away with the *better eye*. (Look 500 ft away if you have moderate myopia. Look 1000 ft away if you have mild myopia.) **Cover** the other eye. Hold the palm 2–3 in. from the eye to prevent instrument myopia. Keep both eyes open. Do the Distance Drill for 30 s.
2. With both lenses still on, look at an object about 500 or 1000 ft away with the *weaker eye*. **Cover** the other eye. Look at the same object in Step 1. Hold the palm 2–3 in. from the eye. Keep both

eyes open. Do the Distance Drill for 30 s. Then take off the lens on the weaker eye.

3. With only the lens on the *better eye*, perform the Snellen Chart Drill. **Cover** the other eye. Hold the palm 2–3 in. from the eye. Keep both eyes open. Stand 5.0 ft away from the chart. Read line 7 five times at a rate of 1 s per letter. Then take the lens off.

4. Insert the lens on the *weaker eye* and perform the Snellen Chart Drill. **Cover** the other eye. Hold the palm 2–3 in. from the eye. Keep both eyes open. Stand 5.0 feet away from the chart. Read line 7 five times at a rate of 1 s per letter. Then take the lens off.

5. Without any lenses on, look outside at an object about 500 or 1000 ft away with *both* eyes. Look at the same object in Step 1. Do the Distance Drill for 1 (one) minute with both eyes. **Not** with each eye separately.

21.8.2   THE MODIFIED PRELIMINARY DRILL TO TREAT SIMPLE ASTIGMATISM OR COMPOUND MYOPIA AND HIGH ASTIGMATISM

1. Wear the lens on the *weaker eye* only. Look outside at an object about 500 ft away. **Do not cover** the other eye that does not have the lens on. Keep both eyes open. Do the distance drill for 30 s.

2. With the lens still on the *weaker eye*, perform the Snellen Chart Drill. **Cover** the other eye. Hold the palm 2–3 in. from the eye. Keep both eyes open. Stand 5.0 ft away from the chart. Read line 7 five times at a rate of 1 s per letter. Then remove the lens.

3. Wear the lens on the *better eye* only. Look at an object about 500 ft away. **Do not cover** the other eye. Look at the same object in Step 1. Keep both eyes open. Do the Distance Drill for 30 s.

4. With the lens still on the *better eye*, perform the Snellen Chart Drill. **Cover** the other eye. Hold the palm 2–3 in. from the eye. Keep both eyes open. Stand 5.0 ft away from the chart. Read line 7 five times at a rate of 1 s per letter. Then remove the lens.

5. Without any lens on, look outside at an object about 500 ft away with the *weaker eye*. **Cover** the other eye. Look at the same object in Step 1. Leave a slight gap 2–3 in. from the eye. Keep both eyes open. Do the Distance Drill for 30 s.

6. Without any lens on, look outside at an object about 500 ft away with the *better eye*. **Cover** the other eye. Look at the same object in Step 1. Leave a slight gap 2–3 in. from the eye. Keep both eyes open. Do the Distance Drill for 30 s.

21.8.3   THE MODIFIED PRELIMINARY DRILL TO TREAT COMPOUND ANISOMETROPIA AND HIGH ASTIGMATISM

1. Wear the lens on the *weaker eye* only. Look outside at an object about 500 ft away. **Do not cover** the other eye that does not have the lens on. Keep both eyes open. Do the Distance Drill for 15 s.
2. With the lens still on the *weaker eye*, perform the Snellen Chart Drill. **Cover** the other eye. Hold the palm 2–3 in. from the eye. Keep both eyes open. Stand 5.0 ft away from the chart. Read line 7 five times at a rate of 1 s per letter. Then remove the lens.
3. Wear the lens on the *better eye* only. Look at an object about 500 ft away. **Do not cover** the other eye. Look at the same object in Step 1. Keep both eyes open. Do the Distance Drill for 15 s.
4. With the lens still on the *better eye*, perform the Snellen Chart Drill. **Cover** the other eye. Hold the palm 2–3 in. from the eye. Keep both eyes open. Stand 5.0 ft away from the chart. Read line 7 five times at a rate of 1 s per letter. Then remove the lens.

KEYWORDS

- **Modified Preliminary Drill**
- **simple astigmatism**
- **corneal astigmatism**
- **lenticular astigmatism**
- **compound astigmatism**

CHAPTER 22

TREATING THE LOSS OF DEPTH PERCEPTION

ABSTRACT

The crystalline lens was not locked in during the onset of myopia. It can still flatten to a certain extent to bring some distant objects into focus. The tension of the oblique muscles does not cause the ciliary muscle to spasm. Instead, it places a restriction on how much the ciliary muscle can relax—and thus how much the lens can flatten out.

The rays of light from near objects are divergent. Wearing a minus lens diverges the light rays even more. The crystalline lens increases its bulged shape to converge the rays onto the retina. The oblique muscles would tighten up some more to alleviate the stress placed on the ciliary muscle. In most cases of moderate myopia, the alleviation is only partial. The result is a partial resistance to ortho C. In severe cases of myopia where the power of the minus lenses is higher, there would be a total resistance. It is the eventual spasm of the ciliary muscle in the attempt to compensate for the longer focal length in the near and midrange that causes a loss of depth perception.

An ortho C lens only attends to the indirect induction of stress—not to any direct induction. Relaxing the oblique muscles by ortho C only deals with the tension of the ciliary muscle that was indirectly induced. If spasticity sets in due to a direct induction of stress, you also have to deal with it separately.

22.1 TIGHTNESS OF THE CILIARY MUSCLE DURING ONSET OF MYOPIA IS NOT ACTUALLY SPASTIC TENSION

Although the ciliary muscle of a myopic eye is tight during onset, it is the excess tension of the oblique muscles that neurologically limits how much the crystalline lens can flatten out for distant focusing. The oblique muscles do not cause the ciliary muscle to spasm. If spasm was induced, it was by some other means—usually by a minus lens. Near-point stress directly induced with a minus lens reduces the ciliary muscle's ability to alternate between tightening up and relaxing to change the shape of the crystalline lens to bring objects at different distances into focus. Objects in front of the eye would be uniformly blurred.

Near-point stress indirectly induced is different. The tension of the oblique muscles places a ceiling on how much the ciliary muscle can relax for distant focusing, but it does not affect the lens' ability to vary its shape within the limitations of the restriction. The ciliary muscle is still flexible enough to allow the lens to assume a bulged shape when the ciliary muscle tenses up during near focusing, and it can still relax to flatten the lens to a certain extent when the eye redirects its attention to something far away.

22.2   LOSS OF DEPTH PERCEPTION AND ITS RELATION TO A MINUS LENS

When a patient became myopic due to near-point stress without any interference from a minus lens, the eye has a lower resistance to ortho C. The assumption is that near-point stress induced by the naked eye is not intense enough to cause the ciliary muscle to spasm when it affects the crystalline lens indirectly. Near-point stress induced by some other means such as constantly wearing a minus lens can cause the ciliary muscle to spasm when it affects the crystalline lens directly.

The light rays from an object in the near range are divergent. If you are looking at it through a minus lens, the light rays would diverge more. The crystalline lens would have to bulge beyond its normal bulged shape to bring the object into focus. The "effort to see" increases when attempting to maintain such a focus. When spasm sets in due to direct induction, the constriction would lock the lens in its maximum bulged shape. As a result, depth perception is compromised as well as distant vision. When the tension of the ciliary muscle was initially due to indirect induction, there was more free play. It was this free play that allowed your patient's depth perception to vary.

22.3   WHY THE EMPHASIS ON THE CILIARY MUSCLE?

If ortho C cannot neurologically activate the ciliary muscle to relax sufficiently to flatten the crystalline lens for distant focusing, the elongated
eyeball would not flatten. The myopic shape of the eyeball can only
"shift" when the lens "shifts." When the lens flattens partially (and cannot
flatten further), the eyeball attempts to alleviate the effort by becoming
less elongated. It is the reverse of near-point stress where the excessive
tension of the ciliary muscle is responsible for the lens bulging as much
as possible, and the eyeball attempts to relieve some of the tension by
assuming an elongated shape.

The application of the Modified Preliminary Drill exemplifies the
theory. The crystalline lens was only partially flattened in Step 1. The
object of regard in Step 2 entices the eyeball to reduce its elongated shape.
The Preliminary Drill cannot duplicate the outcome. The lens flattened too
much in the first part of the drill. It closed the gap between the focal point
and the retina. There is no room to allow the eyeball to follow suit.

22.3.1   LOSS OF DEPTH PERCEPTION IN SEVERE MYOPIA

If the ciliary muscle starts to spasm, the condition falls outside the myopic
model. It diminishes the effectiveness of ortho C. The "contact lens draw"
can directly loosen the oblique muscles, but it cannot deal with the ciliary
muscle's increase in tension. The correct neurological message reinstated
by relaxing the oblique muscles is not sufficient to deal with the excessive
tension directly induced onto the ciliary muscle. The spasm of the ciliary
muscle is a physical as well as a neurological problem. It is not enough to
just reinstate the correct neurological message.

If you wear glasses all the time, you will notice that your surroundings
are uniformly blurred without them. The blanket of blurriness can start just
inches away from you. In some cases of severe myopia, even objects in the
near range (16 in. or 40 cm) would fail to come into focus. It is possible for
everything to be uniformly blur 6 in. away.

Atrophy is another problem that compounds the spasm in the severe
myopic eye. It sets in from disuse when the fixed longer focal length of
a minus lens prohibits the crystalline lens from changing shape. It cannot
participate in distant focusing.

22.3.2   LOSS OF DEPTH PERCEPTION IN MILD AND MODERATE MYOPIA

The patient can still experience a loss of depth perception if the myopia is in the moderate range. The lack of depth perception in the moderate range is different from the severe myopic range. Atrophy may only be partial if the resistance of the eye is partial. The focal length is not as long. A "contact lens draw" may still be able to partially alleviate the tension of the ciliary muscle if the focal point is not too far behind the retina. Although these patients may experience a two-line improvement in visual acuity on the Snellen chart after the first application, there is still a partial loss of vertical depth perception.

22.4   HORIZONTAL AND VERTICAL LOSS OF DEPTH PERCEPTION

When ciliary muscle spasm sets in and produces a state where everything is uniformly blurred the degree of blurriness varies according to the lens power and how often the glasses are worn. It can be measured horizontally and vertically.

The loss of depth perception can be demonstrated horizontally. During the onset of myopia, depth perception is mainly lacking in the distance. Initially, the near range (at 16 in. or 40 cm away) and the midrange or computer range (at 20 in. or 50 cm away) is clear. After the spasm of the ciliary muscle sets in, objects in the near range, in the midrange, and in the distance are equally blurred. It is along a gradient according to the minus lens' power. The spasm of the ciliary muscle and the seizure of the crystalline lens as a result induce the uniform blurriness.

The loss of depth perception can also be demonstrated vertically on a Snellen chart. Prior to the spasm of the ciliary muscle, a moderate myopic eye, for example, may make out the top 3 or 4 lines on the chart clearly with the naked eye, and the lower lines become gradually blur. After the spasm of the ciliary muscle sets in by deciding to wear a pair of glasses all the time, the whole chart in the distance appears uniformly blur.

If a moderate myopic patient disregards the loss of depth perception and proceeds with ortho C, the patient may still experience a two-line improvement on the Snellen chart after the first application, but it would not be as clear as someone without a loss of depth perception. If the client did not have a loss of depth perception and experienced a similar improvement in visual acuity to line 7, for example, the blurriness may start at line 6; but if another the client with a loss of depth perception made a similar gain in visual acuity to line 7, the blurriness would likely start at line 5 or 4.

If your client's prescription is higher, there would be a different scenario. The degree of spasticity inherited by the ciliary muscle can interfere with the "contact lens draw." I have a small percentage of such clients with high myopia who are not responsive to ortho C.

22.5   DEMONSTRATING A LOSS OF DEPTH PERCEPTION

The loss of depth perception can be demonstrated by wearing a pair of minus lenses for extensive reading or computer work after ortho C reduces the refractive error in the moderate to severe range. I did not ask my participants to conduct such a test. Some of my clients accidently wore their weaker glasses to read or to work on the computer. Even though the glasses were undercorrected to allow them to see line 6 or line 7 on the Snellen chart instead of line 8 which is the 20/20 line (to prevent an over-correction outdoors), the focal point is still behind the retina in the near and intermediate range. The crystalline lens would have to bulge to bring an object into focus. During a follow-up, their visual acuity deteriorated by as much as 3 or 4 lines on the Snellen chart.

One participant with severe myopia, for example, had a prescription of -3.00 D and initially experienced good results with ortho C. After a couple of weeks, I tested her with a pair of -1.50 D monthly soft contact lenses. Such a lens simulates a "focal point draw," since the monthly lenses are thicker than the biweekly and daily lenses, and she experienced a visual acuity close to 20/20. Once deterioration set in after she continued to wear her glasses to work on the computer, there was no such response. Besides experiencing a decline in visual acuity with the -1.50 D contact lenses, there was also a reduction in depth perception.

22.6   TEST DEPTH PERCEPTION BEFORE AND AFTER THE DRILL

22.6.1   TEST FOR VERTICAL DEPTH PERCEPTION

Similar to a visual acuity pretest and posttest, check the patient's vertical depth perception before and after performing the assigned drill. It provides information on how much her depth perception has improved as well as her visual acuity. Even if she has a low resistance, the depth perception test can still be conducted. It is possible to have a borderline depth perception and a low resistance.

22.6.1.1   BEFORE THE DRILL

Before conducting the specific drill, ask where the blurriness starts while conducting the v/a test with each eye and with both eyes. If the lines are equally clear, her depth perception is still intact. It is also normal for the blurriness to start at the best line she can see. For example, if she could see down to line 6, line 6 can be slightly blurred, but it is still distinguishable. The chart is clear from line 1 to line 5.

If another patient has a partial resistance, she may also see down to line 6, but the blurriness may start from line 4. Although line 6 is blurred, she can still make it out. It is more blurred, however, than a patient with a low resistance.

If the client cannot tell which line the blurriness starts, then ask if the top half of the chart is clearer than the bottom half or if the top one-third of the chart is clearer than the bottom two-thirds. If the top half of the chart, for example, is clearer than the bottom half, then your client's depth perception is still somewhat intact or partially intact. If only the top two letters are clearer than the rest of the chart, then there is a reduction in depth perception.

22.6.1.2   AFTER THE DRILL

After conducting the specific drill, ask her again which line the blurriness starts after she reads down to the best line (while conducting the v/a test with each eye and with both eyes). If she has a low resistance and could see down to line 8, line 8 can be slightly blurred, but it is still distinguishable. The chart is clear from line 1 to line 7.

22.6.1.3   MENTAL STRAIN AND LOSS OF DEPTH PERCEPTION

I had a participant who was moderately myopic. His prescription was −1.50 D, but he wore his glasses all the time. He did achieve a two-line improvement when he conducted the First Resistance Test, but he would only be aware of it with a weaker prescription. It is difficult for him to notice the improvement with the naked eye due to a loss of depth perception. He depended on his glasses for computer work, and he was reluctant to reduce his wearing time with them in front of the computer screen. He did not like the computer glasses I gave him and preferred to wear the full prescription glasses instead. There is a positive correlation between mental strain and the loss of depth perception.

22.6.2   TEST FOR HORIZONTAL PERCEPTION

You can also check the patient's horizontal depth perception before the drill. There may or may not be a difference afterward because horizontal depth perception is also based on her reading habits in the near and midrange. If she positions herself too close to the object of regard, the habit needs to change. (Refer to the chapter *The Effort to See*.)

Check the degree of horizontal blurriness by having your client sit 50 cm away from a computer screen with a page of text 12 pt Times Romans. Are the letters on the page blurred? Does it clear up more if your client moves into 40 cm? If the letters are blur at 50 cm but clears up at 40 cm, then the midrange depth perception is affected more (the computer range at 20 in. or 50 cm) compared to the near range (the reading range at 16 in. or 40 cm).

I can, for example, read a page of text on the screen 50 cm away as clearly as 40 cm. When working on the computer, I would start at 50 cm away. I would tend to move in closer to the screen after about 5 min. My computer screen is small, and it is comparable to a printed page. I do not work constantly at 50 cm because I am utilizing the maximum flexibility of my lens at that range. Strain would set in if I continue to apply 100% of the flexibility of the lens.

22.6.3   OCULAR MOTILITY TEST

To ensure that the third, fourth, and sixth cranial nerve are transmitting the messages properly to the extraocular muscles, it is a good idea to conduct an ocular test before treating a patient with a partial resistance. Passing the ocular motility test would rule out the comorbidity of other conditions such as Graves disease which can inhibit certain ocular ranges, such as assuming an upward gaze, as well as double vision and blurriness.

To perform the test, have the patient look up and the down vertically. Then look to the upper right and lower left, and then to the upper left and lower right. The eye should also rotate in the direction of gaze. If the patient can perform the test smoothly, then spasticity has not set in.

22.7   THE TREATMENT

Sometimes, there are hints that there is a partial resistance prior to ortho C: the patient's history, the visual acuity test, and/or the patient's constant dependency on glasses. Sometimes, you would not know until you order the lenses and perform the different resistance tests. Even then you would not know until you perform the recommended drill. An eye with a low resistance may still lack the proper depth perception.

In most cases, however, a lack in depth perception correlates with a partial resistance. Ortho C's ability to partially improve an eye that is slightly outside the myopic model indicates that a "contact lens draw" can still relax the tension of ciliary muscle due to indirect stress. The patient still needs to deal with residual loss in depth perception. Ortho C cannot treat the portion of the tension due to direct stress. It was designed to address indirect stress induced by the oblique muscles. The following are some ways to relax the ciliary muscle as much as possible while engaging in ortho C at the same time.

22.7.1   REMOVE THE NEGATIVE VARIABLE BY REMOVING THE GLASSES

If ortho C reinstates the correct neurological message in mild and moderate myopia, you are just treating the indirect stress imposed on the ciliary muscle. That is only one of the stress factors. You still have to deal with any residual direct stress. If those patients continue to rely on their glasses for all distances, for example, it would inhibit any improvement from ortho C. They have to remove the external variable by depending less on their glasses.

Some participants with severe myopia have noticed a partial clarity after a few weeks when they regained part of their depth perception just by relying less on their glasses (or contact lenses). The longer fixed focal length no longer freezes the eye and lens in their myopic shapes. The focal point becomes variable instead of fixed. The focal point of a distant object is in front of the retina. The gap provides some room for the lens to flatten out.

It is possible that the benefit derived from removing the prescription lens' fixed focal point can be partially offset by a jump in "effort to see." It may not immediately occur, but the experience in better vision may trigger it. The increase in effort to see occurs when the partial clarity activates the tendency to increase the clarity or to maintain the clarity without "letting go." The patient needs to realize the moment when the "effort to see" begins to increase. It is an indicator to resort to ortho C before the "effort to see" becomes excessive.

Even after combining some of the following drills just once, such as removing the glasses, palming the eyes, and performing the stretching drill in front of the computer while putting in a full day's work, some of my participants with severe myopia would notice that their visual acuity appears clearer. They may not be able to verify it on the eye chart. There are other subtle signs. When they put their full prescription glasses back on, for example, it would appear too strong.

I would tell them ahead of time to rely on their weaker glasses instead for the distance. The improved visual acuity is due more to the relaxation of the ciliary muscle rather than the relaxation of the oblique muscles. It is more difficult to relax the oblique muscles by just enabling a "focal point draw"—by removing the restriction of a fixed focal length.

A lot of research attempts to treat nearsightedness by reducing the power of the minus lens. The difficulty, however, is that a "focal point draw" must be combined with a "contact lens draw" before the crystalline lens or the eyeball can be influenced to "shift." Otherwise, only the crystalline lens is forced to "shift" on its own accord.

22.7.2 RELY ON MINUS LENSES ONLY FOR THE DISTANCE

It is easier to reduce the reliance on glasses if the myopia is in the mild or moderate range. After the client finish copying notes from the blackboard or from an overhead screen, for example, suggest removing the glasses to avoid a constant exposure to an overcorrection in the near and intermediate range. We spend most of our time in those ranges.

Wearing glasses momentarily for the distance is not as damaging. Light rays 20 ft and beyond reach your eyes as parallel rays. The crystalline lens does not have to bulge that much to bring an object into focus. Light rays closer than 20 ft reach your eye as divergent rays. The closer the object, the more the rays diverge. Wearing a minus lens at the near range diverges the rays even more. The crystalline lens would have to bulge more to converge them to bring an object into focus.

22.7.3   LETTING GO

Explain to the patient the benefits behind adopting the habit of accepting and "letting go" of a blur or a partially blur object instead of straining the eye to bring it into focus. Also, explain how the TV can help. Instead of the TV, watching a movie on a laptop is another option. It trains the patient to "let go" subconsciously instead of continuing to make a conscious effort to bring an object into focus even if it cannot come into focus. The eye learns to adopt an "intermittent draw" instead of a "continuous draw." (Refer to the chapter *Letting Go* and *Addendum* for more information.)

22.7.4   ADJUSTING THE READING AND INTERMEDIATE RANGE

Inform the patient to minimize near-point stress by keep adjusting the reading range until it falls 14–16 in. away to reduce the lens' bulged shape. The patient may not be able to maintain that range, but try to consciously "stretch" and hold it for half a minute or so. Perform the "stretching" drill two or three times a day. After the drill, let the vision settle to its natural range which is a bit closer. Later the patient will be able to adopt the preferred range. The drill is more effective when it is done in conjunction with ortho C.

The same idea applies to working in front of a computer screen. The ideal range in front of a monitor is 20 in. To make the drill more practical, inform the patient to maintain a distance 16–20 in. away depending on the size of the text. (Refer to the chapter *The Effort to See* and to the *Addendum* for more information.)

22.7.5   *RELAXATION EXERCISES*

Explain to the patient the palming and swing drills. Tell the patient to perform the drills regularly, but do not perform them prior to the ortho C drill. Palming, for example, is an extraneous variable because it neurologically interferes with the ortho C drills. (Refer to the *Addendum* for more information.)

22.7.6   *THE 20/20 RULE*

The patient does not have to avoid close-up work to maintain the improvement in visual acuity. Adhering to the 20/20 rule allows the eye to perform the task assigned to it more efficiently. The 20/20 rule states that after 20 min, the patient should take a break by looking away beyond 20 ft for 20 s. A timer can be set at first until it becomes a habit. The patient does not have to look away exactly at 20-min intervals, but he would still look away to relax—even if it is 5 ft away.

22.7.7   *OUTCOME*

Eventually, the improvement in depth perception can unfold as follows: Images close to you will clear up first. Then, the midrange will clear up (your computer distance). An object a bit farther away will not be so clear, and another object farther away will be somewhat blur, etc., as their vision gradually extends to infinity. There is a gradual blurriness in vision along a continuum from near to far. Whereas before, everything before was uniformly blur.

22.7.8   *NO HARM?*

Some eye care specialist would suggest to their patients that there is no harm in wearing a minus prescription when reading extensively. Their arguments were deemed to be reliable since it is possible to duplicate the outcome. For example, if the patient received a new pair of glasses and reads with it extensively for a week, there is no noticeable change in the prescription.

But a phoropter would not immediately pick up a decline in depth perception. It takes longer for your visual acuity to deteriorate. Just because your vision 20 ft away is not immediately affected while reading a test card with your glasses on, it does not mean that your depth perception without your glasses was not compromised.

Our depth perception is affected first, then our visual acuity. How do I know? A specific case study: I allowed my daughter to follow the conventional advice. Her prescription progressed from −1.50 D to −11.50 D. That is her prescription right now at the publication of this book. I did not treat her … yet. It was not intentional. It was due to circumstances. Mind you, back then I did not know what I know now. I just had this theory. I could not prove it. Until now.

KEYWORDS

- depth perception
- spasm
- myopic model
- near-point stress
- direct induction
- indirect induction

CHAPTER 23

TREATING PROGRESSIVE MYOPIA

ABSTRACT

There is a positive correlation between asthenopia (or eye strain) and progressive myopia (or the tendency for one's myopia to become worse). If eye strain is severe, then progressive myopia tends to become worse. Unlike hyperopia, a myopee may not be aware of the progression. The deviation in a hyperopic eye is mainly due to the lens. In the myopic eye, the myopia is due to the eyeball as well as the lens. The eyeball allows extra room for the deviation to set in. It is easier for an excessive "effort to see" to force the crystalline lens and sclera of a myopic eye to become worse almost unnoticed (Yee, 2013b).

Any degree of nearsightedness not only can become worse—but progressively worse. I remember my original pair of glasses was just −0.50 D. At first, I did not wear them all the time, but I was subjected to different types of stress between grade school and high school. My myopia increased rapidly when I started wearing contact lenses. It was not that convenient to take them off when I do not need them for the distance. I was constantly subjected to an overcorrection in the near and midrange. At one point, my prescription deteriorated to −10.00 D. The difficulty with treating higher ranges of myopia lies in the eyeball. It inherits more of the deviation as the myopia gets progressively worse. It is harder to change its curvature compared to the crystalline lens' curvature.

23.1 ASTHENOPIA

Asthenopia, or eye strain, was thought to be prevalent among those with hyperopia (or farsightedness). The symptoms are fatigue, headaches, and blurred vision when performing work in the near range for an extending period. The crystalline lens' inability to take on the proper bulged shape when attempting to bring a near image into focus contributes to the discomfort. Asthenopia is not usually associated with nearsightedness even though the myopia tends to make an effort to bring something far away into focus. The contention is that if the myopic eye cannot make out a blur image, it would eventually give up. The hyperopic eye, on the other hand, would continue trying to bring it into focus.

There may be a correlation, however, between asthenopia and progressive myopia—or the tendency for one's myopia to become worse. Unlike hyperopia, a myopee may not be aware of the progression. The deviation in a hyperopic eye is mainly due to the lens. In the myopic eye, the myopia is due to the eyeball as well as the lens. There is more room for the deviation to set in. (Yee, 2013b).

When the focal point is behind the retina (when the object of regard is close-up), the myopic eye offers less resistance to reposition the focal point onto the retina to bring it into focus. Even if additional stress factors were present to increase the "effort to see," such as dim lighting and wearing a minus lens to read, there is usually the absence of discomfort when progressive myopia sets in. The myopic eye can become progressively myopic almost unnoticed.

23.2   FACTORS INDUCING PROGRESSIVE MYOPIA

Any of the following factors can induce eye strain—which in turn can trigger progressive myopia: an excessive "effort to see," near-point stress, amplified near-point stress, and aggravating factor during development.

23.2.1   EFFORT TO SEE

The habit of making an excessive "effort to see" or maintaining a blur image that temporarily comes into focus can induce eye strain. The brain considers the eye to be in near focus mode due to the excessive tension of the oblique muscles. In that sense, straining to see something far can produce the same symptom as near-point stress.

23.2.2   NEAR-POINT STRESS

The habit of working closer than the recommended distance when working at the near or midrange can induce eye strain. The demands from prolong very near work on the myopic eye (near work closer than 14–16 in. away from the object of regard) can create an excessive "effort to see." Near-point stress can trigger the oblique muscles to tighten up more to allow the sclera to elongate. The tendency for the sclera to elongate reduces the gap between the focal point and the retina to alleviate the ciliary muscle's effort in maintaining the bulged shape of the lens. The tradeoff, however, is that the increase in tension of the oblique muscles can become permanent. The increase in the axial length of the eye can become seized. The extra tension also places more restriction on how much the crystalline lens can flatten for distant focusing.

23.2.3   AMPLIFIED NEAR-POINT STRESS

Wearing a minus lens for the near and intermediate range can also induce eye strain. If it is worn for close-up work, it would be as if though the myopia is inches away from the object of regard. The light rays from a near object are divergent, but a minus lens causes the light rays to diverge even more. It affects the ciliary muscle directly by forcing it to bulge beyond its maximum capacity in the attempt to converge the rays. The excessive effort placed on the ciliary muscle can trigger the oblique muscles to tighten up more to alleviate the tension. Although there is the tendency for the sclera to elongate, it does not immediately alleviate the ciliary muscle's increase in tension due to the wide gap between the focal point and the retina. Thus, the tension on the oblique muscles is progressively tighter.

23.2.4   AGGRAVATING FACTOR DURING DEVELOPMENT

During development, there is a neurological relationship between the crystalline lens and the axial length of the eye—and thus a relationship between the intraocular muscle (the ciliary muscle) and the extraocular muscles (the rectus muscles and the oblique muscles). At birth, the crystalline lens is around +2.00 or +3.00 diopters, and the axial length of the eye is approximately 17 mm. It develops to approximately 24 mm in adulthood.

The "thinning" of the lens occurs at the same time as the increase in the axial length of the eye. The flatness of the lens offsets the elongation of the sclera (or eyeball) to permit proper distant focusing. The changes in the crystalline lens and the axial length of the sclera needs to be synchronized during development to ensure that proper distant focusing is intact. It does not stabilize until the child is around 10 years of age (Mutti et al., 2012).

The tendency for the eyeball to elongate can be thought of as an aggravating factor, and the thinning of the lens in response to the deviation of the eyeball is a compensating factor. When myopia sets in, it further aggravates the eyeball. It already has the tendency to elongate, and near-point stress promotes that tendency. According to Mutti et al. (2012), the lens ceases to compensate for the eyeball once myopia sets in. The crystalline lens would stop "thinning." You would expect that it would start to bulge, but according to Zadnik et al. (1995), the crystalline lens becomes thinner compared to the emmetropic eye.

During near-point stress, the lens displays a lack of a braking mechanism at the near point. Its neutral shape is not round enough. The inability to alleviate the stress directly imposed on the ciliary muscle encourages the eyeball to elongate more than usual. When the lens cannot bulge as much as it should to bring near objects into focus during development compared to postdevelopment, it may account for the increase in the progressive myopia which tends to be more serious at this stage.

There is the question of whether the ciliary muscle responds properly to near focusing even though the lens does not respond properly. According to Oliveira et al. (2005) and Muftuoglu et al. (2009), the ciliary muscle of an adult becomes thicker when it becomes myopic in terms of a longer axial length; and the muscle is thicker compared to the emmetropic eye.

According to Bailey et al. (2008), the ciliary muscle of children is also thicker when they became myopic. In the case of children, there is a different outcome in response to a thicker ciliary muscle. According to Zadnik et al. (1995), the myopic crystalline lens is thinner compared to the emmetropic eye despite the bulged shape of the ciliary muscle. According to Iribarren et al. (2012), an adult myopic lens bulges more compared to the emmetropic eye.

It is easier to treat myopic adults and older teenagers than children. An adult myopic lens behaves as expected in response to a thicker ciliary muscle. It is rounder (or more bulged) during the onset of myopia. There is more room for it to flatten in response to ortho C, since it bulged more compared to the emmetropic eye. When its neutral occluded shape flattens, the eyeball follows suit.

23.3   FACTORS ALLEVIATING ASTHENOPIA

The following factors can alleviate eye strain: compensating factor during postdevelopment, a "contact lens draw," and "focal point draw."

23.3.1   COMPENSATING FACTOR DURING POSTDEVELOPMENT

Barnes (1999) followed a case where progressive myopia did not occurred until adulthood. He gave an example where an individual became mildly myopic during childhood, but he refrained from relying on his glasses unless there was the need to make something out in the distance. He depended on them later as an adult, however, for all ranges of ocular work. His myopia became progressively worse when the minus lenses triggered asthenopia.

After the development stage, there is still a neurological relationship between the crystalline lens and the eyeball. The expected change in the shape of the crystalline lens and eyeball during the postdevelopmental phase is the opposite of the expected changes during the developmental phase. Grosvenor (1987) found that the crystalline lens tends to assume a bulged shape after 20 years of age, and the axial length of the eye decreases to compensate for it. The postdevelopmental stage can be thought of as a later development where the sclera shortens to compensate for the tendency of the crystalline lens to bulge. In this sense, the development of the eye is ongoing during the different phases in the life cycle. The changes ensure that proper distant focusing is maintained.

The tendency for the lens to become rounder can be thought of as an aggravating factor, and the reduction in the axial length of the eye in response to it is a compensating factor. The compensating factor acts as a resistance to progressive myopia. Progressive myopia progresses at a slower rate during postdevelopment compared to the development stage. The tendency for the eye to become shorter from front to back acts as a brake to limit how much it elongates when subjected to near-point stress.

The aggravating factor also offers some resistance to progressive myopia. The tendency for the lens to bulge more compared to the eye during early development alleviates some of the stress inherited by the ciliary muscle. Although the individual may become myopic, there is a better chance for it to be corrected. The lens' flexibility inherited more of the overall nearsightedness. There is more room for the lens to flatten out in response to ortho C. Adolescents and adults seem to exhibit the ideal outcome: the lens would contribute to about 2/3 of the correction, and the eyeball would contribute to about 1/3 of the correction if the eye is in the moderate myopic range.

23.3.2   ORTHO C REVERSES PROGRESSIVE MYOPIA

A "contact lens draw" and "focal point draw" initiate a different relationship between the crystalline lens and sclera. Instead of a rounder crystalline lens stimulating the sclera to elongate due to near-point stress, the "loosening" of the oblique muscles stimulates a flatter crystalline lens. A flatter occluded neutral shape of the lens stimulates the sclera to shorten for distant focusing. The loosening of the oblique muscles simultaneously tightening the rectus muscles to enable the sclera to shorten. The reduction in the myopic shape of the sclera neurologically triggers it to synchronize with the lens according to a postdevelopment relationship.

23.4   THE TREATMENT

The drill for dealing with progressive myopia depends on the resistance of the eye. The level of resistance is determined by the resistance tests. Each level is an indication of the eye's flexibility and thus which drill to adopt. In addition to performing the drill, you have to find what is contributing to progressive myopia. The tension of the ciliary muscle becomes progressively tighter if the induced tension was maintained. One of the ways it becomes tighter is by wearing a minus lens in the near and midrange. If spasticity sets in, the eye may put up a total resistance to ortho C instead of a partial resistance.

You have to educate your clients on the concept of having to see a bit worse to allow for some free play between the focal point and the retina by relying less on their minus lenses. In the process, they have to "let go" of making an effort to see clear all the time. They have to learn to accept a blur image in the distance (as explained in the chapter *Letting Go*). They should also strive to maintain the proper reading and computer range to prevent the ciliary muscle from become too tense. The proper reading range is 14–16 in., and the proper computer range is 16–20 in. They also have to relax their eyes to relieve the spasm of the ciliary muscle. (Refer to the chapter *The Effort to See* and the *Addendum* for more information.) They need to adopt those habits to halt the progression before ortho C can be effective. According to Lally et al. (2010), a new habit can be created by repeating it enough times (about 66 times). (Refer to the chapter *The Effort to See* for more information.)

KEYWORDS

- asthenopia
- effort to see
- near-point stress
- amplified near-point stress
- development
- postdevelopment
- aggravating factor

CHAPTER 24

WEARING SCHEDULE

ABSTRACT

You have to wear the lenses regularly. The oblique muscles can become tight again when left unattended. In the short term, the wearing schedule is more frequent. Afterwards, the interval becomes longer. The main reason for relying less and less on the ortho C lenses is to allow the crystalline lens and eyeball to synchronize in each eye and to allow one eye to synchronize with the other. The specific drill attends to the first and second myopic relationship. By relying less on the lenses and the drill, it attends to the third and fourth myopic relationship.

Just like adhering to a maintenance schedule after shedding some excess weight, your client also needs to maintain the improvement in vision. The oblique muscles can become tight again when left unattended. By adhering to a maintenance schedule, you are addressing the tendency for myopia to progress as well as its present state. The phenomenon is common in laser surgery. There is still the tendency for the oblique muscles to increase their tension and induce a partial relapse. The initial excessive tension was not attended to during the treatment.

24.1 DIFFERENCE BETWEEN A LOW RESISTANCE EYE AND A PARTIAL RESISTANCE EYE

The following are some differences between a low resistance eye (within the myopic model) and an eye with a partial resistance (outside the myopic model):

- A low resistance eye can improve by 2–3 lines on the Snellen chart after performing the recommended drill just once.

- A partial resistance eye can only improve by 2 lines or less after performing the recommended drill just once. In some cases, it may also exhibit an improvement of 2–3 lines, but it lacks depth perception.
- A patient with a low resistance who sees down to line 8 with the naked eye, for example, may experience that line as slightly blur, but line 7 is clear.
- A patient with a partial resistance may also see down to line 8 with the naked eye and may also experience that line as slightly blur, but the blurriness may extend to line 5. The loss of vertical depth perception is wider.
- A low resistance eye can immediately start in extending its retention period.
- A partial resistance eye needs to go through a different process to relax the ciliary muscle before it can extend its retention period.

24.2   WEARING SCHEDULE FOR THE LOW RESISTANCE EYE

24.2.1   DETERMINING THE PROPER RETENTION PERIOD FOR THE SHORT AND MEDIUM TERM

The retention period is the period from the day the drill maximizes the improvement in visual acuity to the day when the visual acuity starts to falter. Before you attempt to extend the retention period of an eye with a low resistance, have the client perform the recommended drill two times a week for 1 week. Then ask the patient to monitor how long the improved visual acuity would last. If the retention is less than a week, the patient would perform the drill again just once along with the relaxation exercises mentioned in the *Addendum*. The patient would again check the visual acuity daily to find how long the improved visual acuity would last.

The improvement in visual acuity does not wear off completely after a certain period. For example, there may be a slight drop in depth perception. If the client sees line 8 and the blurriness starts at line 7, the blurriness may start from line 5 or line 6 after a week. He may still see line 8, but the blurriness starts to widen its gap. Once the gap extends beyond a certain range, there would be a regression of a line on the chart. To ensure a progressive retention, the patient should perform the drill again before the regression stabilizes.

If the retention lasts for a week, for example, then the wearing schedule is once a week. You would adhere to that schedule until the retention period becomes longer. If it extends to a week and a half, then the wearing schedule becomes a week and a half, etc. Keep in mind that each time the retention period increases, it may take longer before the patient experiences the next increase. The goal is to extend the retention period to about a month.

If the eye is very flexible, it may gain an improvement in retention immediately. It may also achieve maximum retention without the patient being aware of it. For example, the patient's retention period may be 3 weeks. After performing the drill again, it may extend its retention by another 3 days. The patient may not be aware of the incremental increase in retention.

An eye with a primary refractive error within the myopic model tends to have the longest retention period. It is followed by an eye with a secondary refractive error within the myopic model. There is the tendency for an eye with compound anisometropia and anisometropic amblyopia to acquire a longer retention period than an anisometropic eye. A myopic or anisometropic eye and high astigmatism ranks last. It is not just a matter of establishing the correct neurological message. There is also the task of realigning the mismatch in the tension of the rectus muscles.

If there is no improvement in retention, check if the patient is overly sensitive to the lenses, if there is an increase in resistance due to mistakes, or if there are any negative offsetting factors. Ensure that the recommended drill matches the specific problem. Also check that you calculated the flatness factor properly. For other problems, refer to the chapter *Troubleshooting*.

24.2.2   PROGRESSIVE RETENTION AND LINEAR RETENTION

The patient should find the retention period lasting a bit longer each time the drill is performed. The duration tends to exceed the previous retention period. If it does, the duration is progressive. If the retention is about the same over an extended period, the duration is linear.

At some point, the progressive retention will peak. There are usually only two or three consecutive increases in retention in the short to medium term. The short term is within 1 month, and the medium term is within 3 months. When it peaks, that would be the wearing schedule for that term. For example, after the patient performed the drill again, you found that the retention period is still 3 weeks. If it was like that for the last few sessions, then that is the wearing schedule. The patient would perform the drill once every 3 weeks.

It is a good idea to perform the relaxation drills to relax the ciliary muscle now and then. It makes a difference between an eye stuck in linear retention and an eye whose retention increases progressively. You also have to minimize any stress directly induced by adhering to the proper distance when working at the near or midrange. (Refer to the *Addendum* for more information.)

24.2.3 THE EXTENDED RETENTION PERIOD

The main reason why the patient relies less and less on the lenses is to allow the crystalline lens and eyeball to synchronize in each eye and to allow one eye to synchronize with the other. The specific drill attends to the first and second myopic relationship. By relying less on the lenses and the drill, it attends to the third and fourth myopic relationship. An increase in the retention period can continue to the point where some patients do not rely on a fixed schedule. Sometimes, they would notice that their visual acuity starts to waver a bit after about 3 months. Sometimes it is after 4 months. It depends on the exposure to near work and to the computer monitor. If the eye has a low resistance and if the mild or moderate myopic eye is within the myopic model, its extended retention rivals laser surgery.

24.3 WEARING SCHEDULE FOR THE PARTIAL RESISTANCE EYE

24.3.1 DETERMINING THE PROPER RETENTION PERIOD FOR THE SHORT AND MEDIUM TERM

Before you attempt to extend the retention period of an eye with a partial resistance, have the client perform the recommended drill two or three times a week for 2 weeks—along with the relaxation exercises mentioned in the *Addendum*, but do not perform the relaxation exercises and the specific drill at the same time. After 2 weeks, ask the patient to monitor how long the improved visual acuity would last after the last drill. If the retention is less than a week, the patient would perform the drill two or three times a week for another 2 weeks along with the relaxation exercises. If the retention is still less than a week, the patient would then perform the drill just once a week while relying on the relaxation exercises more often. It gives the crystalline lens and eyeball a chance to synchronize. The third myopic relationship should also be given an opportunity to reverse by allowing the postdevelopmental relationship of the lens and eyeball to reestablish.

24.3.2   LAG IN RETENTION PERIOD

The eye's progressive retention tends to lag behind the low resistance eye in the short and medium term. In the moderate myopic eye with a partial resistance, the eyeball may have deviated more. It takes a bit longer for the eyeball to retract. If the crystalline lens bulged more, it is easier to reverse; but if the eyeball deviated more, the reversal may require physiotherapy as well as resetting the correct neurological message. Some relaxation exercises may be required to relax the ciliary muscle. The patient performs the relaxation drills mentioned in the *Addendum* to relax the partial spasm of the ciliary muscle. The rectus muscles increase their strength by flexing and letting go whenever the patient wears the lenses and removes them. It works together with the relaxed ciliary muscle in reversing the myopic eyeball.

24.3.2.1   VISUAL ACUITY TEST

Conduct a visual acuity test regularly. Check with the weaker glasses as well as with the naked eye. The weaker glasses relax the ciliary muscle to give a more accurate reading. The naked eye may fluctuate when reading the chart due to an increase in "effort to see." Often an improvement in visual acuity is more noticeable with the glasses on than with the naked eye when there is a partial resistance. (Refer to the chapter *The Procedure* for more information.)

24.3.2.2   ADJUST THE INDICATOR

Glasses tend to be better indicator for an improvement in visual acuity instead of the naked eye. When there is an improvement in visual acuity with the weaker glasses to allow line 9 or 10 to come into focus, you have to issue another pair of glasses that allows only line 7 to come into focus again, etc. The ability to see line 9 or 10 under normal conditions is an indication of the patient's night vision. That pair of glasses would be kept in the vehicle for night driving. There is a lack of a "focal point draw" at night when the aperture of the eye opens wider. A pair of glasses allowing the patient to see line 7 in adequate indoor lighting (where you hanged the eye chart) would be more than adequate for driving in the daytime. (Refer to the section on *Visual Acuity Test* in the *Addendum* for more information.)

24.3.3   ESTABLISH THE PROPER RETENTION PERIOD IN THE LONG TERM

The long-term goal is to stimulate the eye to adopt a progressive retention cycle. How long it would take to break out of the partial resistance mode depends on the type of resistance as well as the degree of resistance. A compound astigmatic eye with a high cylinder is an indication of a partial resistance eye. It can break out of the mode immediately if it is within the myopic model. It takes longer to break out of the mode if it is slightly outside the myopic model.

It also depends on the patient's commitment to adhere to the wearing schedule. The maximum retention period takes a longer time to determine compared to the low resistance eye. Some of my participants with a partial resistance are content with a linear retention period. They wear the lenses regularly and perform the recommended drill to maintain the level of retention. If they cannot see the blackboard, they would just wear the weaker glasses.

They continue with the wearing schedule with the expectation that they would benefit in the long term. They also perform the relaxation drills regularly to relax the ciliary muscle and minimize any stress directly induced by adhering to the proper distance when working at the near or midrange as outlined in the *Addendum*. At some point, I may suggest that they break away from the weekly wearing schedule and not perform the drill for a couple of weeks and see what happens. From my experience in dealing with higher myopic ranges, some participants reported seeing better after an extended break.

24.4   WHY STRIVE TO WEAR THE LENS LESS AND LESS?

To prevent fatigue, do not perform the recommended drill for more than once a day and do not perform it every day. It is not like ortho K where the longer you wear the lenses, the better. The frequency of wear is the opposite. The intention is to reduce your dependency on them. The flatness factor was designed according to the patients' original prescription prior to ortho C—not according to their improved visual acuity. Once their vision has improved as much as possible, the oblique muscles are not that tense. The "contact lens draw" becomes excessive if you keep applying a "focal point draw" when it is not necessary—such as when the eye becomes emmetropic. The approach in maintaining their improved visual acuity is not to wear the lenses more frequently. It is the opposite. The goal is to wear the lenses less.

The oblique muscles need to tighten up slightly before performing the drill again. If the oblique muscles are still relaxed (after performing the drill), there is no need to reestablish the correct neuromuscular message. It is not a good idea to keep initiating the correct neurological message when it is not required. It may inadvertently force some part of the eye to change when it had not deviated. It is like forcing the emmetropic lens or sclera to become less elongated when it is not necessary to do so. The visual acuity would become blur.

The patient needs to find the duration when the increase in tension starts to occur. The muscles would not become as tight as they were prior to ortho C. The slight tension would start to increase the gap between the focal point and the retina. The patient would notice some fluctuation in different settings such as outdoors versus indoors. It is an indication that it is time to do the drill again.

Spacing out the drill appropriately allows the synchronization between the crystalline lens and eyeball to take place—assuming your client is in the postdevelopmental stage. During postdevelopment, the eyeball needs to flatten to compensate for the tendency for the crystalline lens to bulge. Eventually, you want the postdevelopmental relationship to assist in the retention of your client's improved visual acuity. You may interrupt that relationship if you keep resetting the neurological message.

KEYWORDS

- **retention period**
- **low resistance**
- **partial resistance**
- **progressive retention**
- **linear retention**

PART 3
Verification

CHAPTER 25

REINSTATING THE CORRECT MESSAGE

ABSTRACT

The first part of the book specified that the myopic eye responds better to ortho C if there are no signs of any extraneous variables. Besides the myopic eye, an extraneous variable can also affect the proposed drills and the design of the lens. In this chapter, I am basing the success of the treatment on the reliability of the ortho C lens by emphasizing its standard design and on arguments why the outcome is due to neurology. I also suggested an experiment to demonstrate that if you deviated from standardization, ortho C would not work. (In the next chapter, I will provide verification on the method.)

Verification starts with examining the apparatus. I want to demonstrate that an ortho C lens does not inadvertently alter the cornea directly after removal; otherwise, the lens would not be able to do what it was designed to do. I also want to demonstrate that precise measurements in its design are necessary to reduce the tension of the oblique muscles by a specific amount before the motor cortex can reset the correct neurological message. If the lens' thickness is outside the allowable tolerance, for example, ortho C would not work properly.

Furthermore, I want to demonstrate that the treatment involves neurology. An ortho C lens stimulates the eye directly by creating a "contact lens draw" to loosen the oblique muscles. It triggers a "focal point draw" when the correct message is relayed to the ciliary and rectus muscles. When the multiplier effect flattens the crystalline lens, it reverses the first myopic relationship; and when the multiplier effect reduces the elongated shape of the eyeball at the same time, it reverses the second myopic relationship.

Besides the above demonstrations, I am also including a formal demonstration at the end of the chapter. You can duplicate the experiment to prove that ortho C reinstates the correct neurological message. The correct message depends on the proper "contact lens draw" which in turn depends on the thickness of the lens.

25.1   THE APPARATUS

25.1.1   IT DOES NOT FLATTEN THE CORNEA

There is the contention that the lens may flatten the curvature of the cornea after removing the lens, and it is the flatter cornea that contributes to good vision—not the modified shape of the crystalline lens or the sclera. Although an ortho C contact lens is slightly flatter than the cornea, the intention is not to "push" against the cornea but to produce a "contact lens draw." You want to avoid wearing an ortho C lens too long. It would simulate an ortho K lens by pushing against the cornea instead of drawing on it after the solution drains, but ortho C and ortho K do not mix.

I can demonstrate that ortho K activates a neurological message which is not compatible with ortho C by changing the standard thickness of an ortho C lens to the standard thickness of a conventional rigid gas permeable (RGP) lens—by changing a lens from 0.15 to 0.18 mm. Just by altering this specification, it simulates an ortho K lens. It would not "draw" on the eye but would push against it. By performing the same drill just once, your patient's improved visual acuity (from engaging in ortho C) would deteriorate.

The patient only had the lens on for a few minutes—not hours. It is unlikely that an ortho C lens can alter the curvature of the cornea in such a short period. The flatness of an ortho C lens fitted for mild and moderate myopia is only a fraction of the flatness of an ortho K lens. If the prescription is −0.50 D for both eyes, the flatness of the lens is 0.50 D. An overnight ortho K lens can be as flat as 6.0 D to treat myopia up to −6.00 D. Even with that degree of flatness, the cornea cannot retain the modified shape immediately. When it does assume that shape by wearing the lens overnight, the cornea would start to deteriorate after a day or two. With ortho C, the outcome is the opposite. The retention is immediate, and it lasts much longer.

The contention that a partially flat ortho C lens can still induce a flatter cornea can be addressed by pointing out that the flatness of a conventional RGP lens can be from 0.25 D to 1.00 D flatter than the cornea. It is already according to standard practice that a conventional RGP lens is made flatter for a better fit due to the unevenness of the cornea. Its thickness is 0.18 mm. It is not as flexible as an ortho C lens, but the assumption is that the curvature of the cornea does not change. Otherwise, it would alter the tear layer which is included in the calculation for the power of the lens.

According to common practice, a conventional RGP lens is made flatter than the lower or flatter curve. An ortho C lens' curvature is flatter than mid K: the curve between the top or steeper curve and the bottom or the flatter curve. In that respect, an ortho C lens can be less flat than a conventional RGP lens given the myopic range it was designed to treat.

An ortho C lens is definitely not as flat as an ortho K lens, and the patient only wears the lenses for a few minutes. You can verify that the cornea does not change by taking a K reading before and afterward. If the cornea did not change but the patient sees better, then something else in the eye was altered.

25.1.2   IT IS NOT DUE TO THE TEAR FACTOR

Although the ortho C lenses are a plain pair of lenses, your client will actually see better with them on. The improvement in vision is often attributed to the "tear factor" or the "tear layer" rather than to a change in the crystalline lens or sclera. An ortho C lens' curvature is slightly flatter, and it creates a gap between the lens' flange and the cornea. The contention is that the contact lens solution would fill the gap to take on the shape of a minus lens. It refracts the rays of light that meet the lens. The parallel rays from a distant image would diverge to project its focal point closer to the retina. The effect is similar to wearing a minus lens.

However, you can see through an instrument called a slit lamp that the edge of an ortho C lens adheres closer to the cornea compared to a conventional hard contact lens with a similar flatness. An ortho C lens is 0.15 mm thick instead of 0.17 or 0.18 mm thick (which is the standard thickness of a conventional "plano" lens). The meniscus minimizes the gap between the contact lens and the cornea. Thus, it also minimizes the effect of the tear layer.

The tear factor contributes to some of the clarity in visual acuity while you have the lenses on, but it does not account for the degree of improvement that you experience when you take the lens off. If the moderately myopic eye is receptive, it is possible to see a two- or three-line improvement on the Snellen chart after one application (after wearing the lenses for about 5 min). More importantly, the ability to permanently retain your improvement in vision in such a short time after you remove the lenses cannot be due to the tear factor.

25.2   THE MEASUREMENTS

25.2.1   THE PROPER THICKNESS

An ortho C lens must be 0.15 mm thick. If you designed a plain contact lens with the proper flatness but with a slight increase in its thickness, such as 0.18 mm, your client's visual acuity would remain unchanged after performing the recommended drill. Since the lens is 0.18 mm thick, it is not flexible enough to produce a "contact lens draw." You are applying ortho K—not ortho C.

25.2.2   THE PROPER FLATNESS FACTOR

If you do not abide by the specifications for the flatness factor as outlined in the chapter *Specifications* and instead chose a very flat lens, such as 2.00 D, to deal with mild myopia, the immediate improvement in vision would be due to the tear factor. Once you remove the lens, the client would no longer experience the clarity. The "contact lens draw" was incorrect even if the thickness of the lens is correct. Another interesting phenomenon is that if you had improved the patient's visual acuity with the correct ortho C lens prior to wearing the flatter lens, the improvement would be reduced or erased.

Suppose the patient's prescription was OD −1.50 D and OS −1.50 D and ortho C maximized the improvement in visual acuity. A change in the flatness of the lens by even 0.50 D would cause blurriness to set in. If you increase the flatness of the lenses to 2.00 D for example, it is possible for the patient to see less by 2 or 3 lines. The deterioration only took a few minutes. You initiated a different neurological message. It either altered a part of the eye that does not need to be changed, or it was altered more than how much it deviated. The eye cannot maintain the altered shape.

25.2.3   CORRECTING ONLY THE PART (OR PARTS) OF THE EYE THAT DEVIATED

An ortho C lens should only attend to the part of the eye that is responsible for the refractive error. If your patient's prescription is −0.50 D, then the crystalline lens and sclera need to be "flatten" by 0.50 D to offset the deviation. The restriction placed on the ciliary muscle by the spasm of the oblique muscles has to be lowered by 0.50 D. You need a lens with a flatness of 0.50 D not to flatten the cornea but to relax the tension of the oblique muscles by that amount. It would not just relax the tension of the ciliary muscle but also increase the tension of the rectus muscles.

If instead you designed a lens with a flatness of 2.00 D with just the intention of shortening the eyeball, it would not correct the refractive error. The intention may be logical. If the eye's axial length becomes less, it can enhance your vision by bringing the focal point of a distant image closer to the retina; but it implies reversing a part of the eye that was not myopic. The eyeball would not have deviated by that much. The assumption is that the eyeball only deviated slightly with a prescription of −0.50 D. Most of the myopia is inherited by the lens.

Ortho C is a reversal process. It reverses only the part (or parts) of the eye that became myopic. To reverse the mild myopic eye back to its premyopic shape, the crystalline lens needs to "shift" more than the eyeball. If the globe of the eye retained its spherical shape, then it does not need to be altered. If you insist on flatten it, you are not reversing its myopic shape; you are modifying its normal shape. It would be similar to altering the shape of an emmetropic eye. Instead of resetting the proper neurological message, you are changing it. If you change the proper neurological message, you may end up seeing blur.

25.2.4   CORRECTING ONLY WITHIN THE RANGE OF DEVIATION

An ortho C lens should only reverse the deviated part of the eye within its range of deviation. If an ortho C lens attempts to flatten the myopic crystalline lens excessively, the patient may see better at first; but there is the tendency for the lens to revert back to its myopic bulged shape. If you force the crystalline lens to change its shape by 2.00 D when your prescription was only −0.50 D, for example, you are not reinstating the neuromotor message to reset the curvature of the crystalline lens. You are attempting to change the shape of the crystalline lens beyond its deviation. The modified shape would not hold.

25.3   NEUROLOGICAL ASPECTS OF THE TREATMENT

25.3.1   NEUROLOGICAL COMPONENT BEHIND THE SPECIFICATIONS

There is a neurological component in the treatment related to the measurements. If the lens is not flat enough, the treatment is not optimal. If the lens is flatter than the maximum flatness allowed according to the Flatness Factor chart, ortho C will not work. You cannot overcorrect the patient's myopia. You can only correct the lens or eyeball within the deviated range. To demonstrate the theory, if you place a lens 0.50 D flatter on an emmetropic eye, the eye will become myopic. Objects in the distance will become blurred.

You cannot alter any parts of an eye that had not deviated. It would take too much effort to maintain the new shape. The rectus muscles would have to tighten up more than what is normally required, and the oblique muscles would have to "loosen" beyond their capacity. There is the tendency for those muscles to revert back to their former shapes to alleviate that effort.

25.3.2   INDIRECT INFLUENCE

If the patient just had one lens on while performing the Distance Drill, there is an indirect influence on the other eye. How do you explain the improved visual acuity of the other eye not wearing the lens? And why does it improve even when that eye was occluded? It cannot be due to a mechanical influence (Yee, 2011).

25.3.3   THE ABILITY TO DISCRIMINATE AMONG THE DIFFERENT TYPES OF TREATMENT

The reinstatement of the correct neurological message is also evident when the motor cortex selects the right treatment among the various refractive errors. An ortho C lens is not designed differently to treat mild myopia and the different types of simple astigmatism that fall within the same dioptric range. The lens' flatness is identical, for example, when treating one patient with mild myopia of −0.50 D and another patient with simple astigmatism of −0.50 D.

To correct mild myopia, the lens "stretches" the oblique muscles by 0.50 D to allow the crystalline lens to flatten out uniformly for distant focusing (Yee, 2011). To correct lenticular astigmatism, it "stretches" the oblique muscles by 0.50 D to allow the crystalline lens to flatten along a specific meridian for distant focusing (Yee, 2013a). And to correct corneal astigmatism, it "stretches" the oblique muscles by 0.50 D to allow the crystalline lens to compensate for the distortion of the cornea along a specific meridian (Yee, 2012). The improvement in visual acuity is not totally due to the design of the ortho C lens. It did not differentiate between correcting the crystalline lens due to mild myopia or to the different types of simple astigmatism. It was designed only to relax the oblique muscles. It is the brain's motor cortex that fine-tunes the correction after the oblique muscles are relaxed sufficiently.

25.3.4   TREATING REFRACTIVE ERRORS OTHER THAN MILD OR MODERATE MYOPIA

In other instances, the design of the lens is problem specific. There are exceptions to the specifications mentioned in the Flatness Factor. Those specifications are intended to treat mild and moderate myopia with a low resistance. There are other refractive errors such as anisometropia and high astigmatism that offer a slightly higher resistance. They are still treatable. Although they have a partial resistance, they are still within the myopic model.

The chapter *The Procedure* gives a list of conventional drills for different refractive errors. It also gives another list of alternative drills when the conventional drills do not apply. It does not mean the conventional drills are ineffective. The alternative drills address an eye with a partial resistance due to an extraneous variable. It caused a primary refractive error to deviate outside the myopic model.

25.3.5   REVERSING THE FIRST AND SECOND MYOPIC RELATIONSHIP

When an ortho C lens relaxes the oblique muscles, the motor cortex relays a message to reverse the first myopic relationship between the oblique muscles and the ciliary muscle to allow the crystalline lens to flatten. The relaxation of the oblique muscles also relays a message to reverse the second myopic relationship between the oblique muscles and the rectus muscles to allow the eye to retract. The outcome is the opposite of near-point stress.

25.4   AN EXPERIMENT

A formal experiment can be conducted to demonstrate that it is the "contact lens draw" that triggers an improvement in visual acuity. Although the "draw" depends on the flatness factor as well as the thickness, the contact lens' thickness needs to be more exact than its flatness before a "draw" is possible. If the thickness is off by 0.02 mm, ortho C would not work; but if the flatness is slightly off, it may still work. For example, if you apply a flatness factor of 0.50 D to treat an eye with a prescription of OU −1.00 D, the results would not be optimum, but it would still work. The margin of error is wider.

The participants are separated into two groups: an experimental group and a control group. There are four participants in each group with moderate myopia. You would ask about their history to rule out the presence of any extraneous variables. The following are the prescription of each participant in the experimental group: −1.00 D, −1.25 D, −1.50 D, and −1.75 D. It is similar to the prescription of each participant in the control group: −1.00 D, −1.25 D, −1.50 D, and −1.75 D. The prescription for the right and left eye is the same.

In both groups, you would design the participants' RGP lenses with a flatness factor equal to the absolute value of the prescription. In the experimental group, the thickness of the lenses is 0.15 mm. In the control group, the lenses have a standard thickness of 0.18 mm.

Each participant conducts the Standard Drill. You would check the visual acuity of each participant afterward. You would find that there is only an improvement in visual acuity in the experimental group.

The flatness and tear factor are similar in both groups. The only difference is the thickness. There is no "contact lens draw" in the control group since a lens with a thickness of 0.18 mm is not flexible enough to produce a "contact lens draw" Thus, the improvement in visual acuity in the experimental group is due to a "contact lens draw," since a thickness of 0.15 mm allows the lens to be flexible enough to enable a "contact lens draw."

KEYWORDS

- apparatus
- cornea
- tear factor
- thickness
- flatness factor
- deviation
- ortho K

CHAPTER 26

FOLLOW-UPS

ABSTRACT

In the previous chapter, verification is in reference to the apparatus. In this chapter, verification is in reference to the method. During a follow-up, the main emphasis is to ensure that the patient follows the instructions for the specific drill. The ability to maintain the benefits gained from ortho C by adhering to protocol demonstrates the standardization in the treatment.

In the medical profession as well as in optometry, only a few follow-ups are permitted free of charge. I decided to try something outrageous. What if I did not place a limit on the number of follow-ups? With that policy in mind, I found that even the most concerned participants would only visit me, on average, up to about eight times before they are comfortable. They would see me perhaps once every 2 weeks at first. Once they are satisfied that everything is according to expectation, then the schedule becomes a monthly or quarterly arrangement. Even then I would not charge them. It makes good business sense. They would often refer other participants to me. The goal is to enable the patients to become independent—to rely on you less. Once they reached that level, then you want them to rely on the lenses less. It involves a learning process and that is another reason to extend the follow-ups. You do not want to force them to become independent before they are ready.

26.1 CHECK THE PATIENT'S VISUAL ACUITY

Check the patient's visual acuity with and without any visual aid. Check if the v/a is close to the v/a you took during the last follow-up. If there is a difference, why? Is the patient taking advantage of the weaker glasses, or did he resort back to the stronger glasses? Did the client depend on prescription contact lenses just once or twice to play sports? Wearing soft contacts just a few times is enough to cause a partial resistance even if those contacts were undercorrected. How often did the client perform the drill? Was it performed at all since the last visit?

Check for a loss of depth perception during a v/a test. If the client sees line 8, the 20/20 line, the story does not end there. If it is slightly blur, where does the blurriness start? If it from line 7, it is acceptable; but if it starts at line 4 or 5, you corrected the visual acuity but not the depth perception. Perhaps a negative offsetting factor crept in. To address the loss of depth perception, refer to the chapter *Treating the Loss of Depth Perception*.

If the patient was engaged in the Preliminary Drill instead of the Standard Drill to get used to the ortho C lenses, some fluctuation is acceptable; but it should not regress to its original prescription. If the patient's binocular visual acuity had improved to line 8 from line 5 during the initial visit, a change in focus down to line 7 during a follow-up is acceptable—or even down to line 6. The patient should switch over to the Standard Drill before a resistance builds up.

After performing the Standard Drill a few times, there should hardly be any fluctuation binocularly. If there is some fluctuation, it may be related to the weaker eye. The better eye maintains the clarity, and it determines the binocular vision.

26.2   IF THE PATIENT ADOPTED BAD HABITS

If the patient adopted any bad habits such as squinting, reading too close, etc., you want to ensure that he dealt with the problem. (Refer to the chapter *The Effort to See* for more information.) Ask if he followed the 20/20 rule and the relaxation, swinging, and stretching drills as outlined in the *Addendum*. You also want to ensure that there are no other offsetting variables.

26.3   IF THE PATIENT HAD A PARTIAL RESISTANCE

If the patient had a partial resistance to ortho C, check if he broke out of the partial resistance mode. After performing the wearing schedule two or three times a week for 2 weeks, check his retention. Ask if he followed the 20/20 rule and the relaxation, swinging, and stretching drills as outlined in the *Addendum*. (Refer to the chapter *Wearing Schedule* for more information on extending the retention period.)

26.4   ATTEMPT THE ACTUAL DRILL

If the patient was practicing only with the first part of the Preliminary Drill for a couple of weeks to adapt to the contact lenses, you may want to encourage him to try the actual drill, such as the Standard Drill, during the second follow-up. The results from the Standard Drill produce another "shock" that is more intense in addressing a primary refractive error than the results from the Preliminary Drill. The client would often be surprise to find the outcome equivalent to laser surgery if the eye has a low resistance. Unlike the Preliminary Drill, the results from the Standard Drill should display hardly any fluctuation.

26.5   CHECK THE MEASUREMENTS AND PROCEDURES

Ensure that the patient adheres to the measurements in the specific drill. For example, the patient must stand 5.0 ft from the Snellen chart, and line 7 is the lowest line the patient should read regardless if it is possible to make out the lower lines, the letters are read at a rate of one second per letter, etc.

Also ensure that the patient adheres to the procedures. For example, in some drills, the lens for the weaker eye is worn first; and in other drills, the lens for the better eye is worn first. In some drills, both lenses are worn in the first part of the drill; in other drills, only one lens is worn individually in the first part of the drill.

I found that some participants with anisometropia are more sensitive to any changes in protocol. One of them told me that it was very strenuous when she inadvertently did the Distant Drill beyond 500 ft. Another participant with anisometropic amblyopia noticed a drastic decline in visual acuity when she accidentally mixed up the lenses.

26.5.1   THE PRELIMINARY DRILL

If the patient was practicing the Preliminary Drill at home, check how he performs it at the clinic. Check that he wears the lenses one at a time in the first part of the drill. He does not cover the other eye. The second part of the drill is essentially the same as the Standard Drill. The lenses are worn one at a time, and the other eye is covered. The exception is that the wearing sequence is different from the Standard Drill. Check that he does not wear any lenses in the last part of the drill.

26.5.2   THE STANDARD DRILL

If the patient was practicing the Standard Drill at home, check how he performs it at the clinic. Check that he wears both lenses together only in the first part of the drill. He keeps both eyes opened even though he covers one eye. The second part of the drill is essentially the same as the Preliminary Drill. The lenses are worn one at a time, and the other eye is covered. The exception is that the wearing sequence is different from the Preliminary Drill. Check that he does not wear any lenses in the last part of the drill.

26.5.3   THE MODIFIED PRELIMINARY DRILL

If the patient was practicing the Modified Preliminary Drill at home, check how he performs it at the clinic. Similar to the Preliminary Drill, the lenses are worn one at a time. The exceptions are that the supplementary drills are performed together for each eye, and the last two steps of the Modified Preliminary Drill to treat astigmatism are not included when treating anisometropia.

26.6   CHECK IF THE PATIENT IS EXPERIMENTING

Some patients may have biases and preconceived notion on how to treat myopia. They may want to experiment with the guidelines. I suggest you ask the question, "Have you performed the drill according to the steps I gave you?" (Assuming you gave them a copy of the steps involved.) You have to ask the question directly instead of alluding to it. Ask if they followed the procedures exactly instead of asking if the steps were performed properly. Sometimes there is the notion that any alteration is deemed to be proper. If they mentioned they followed the procedures, then ask a variation of the following just in case, "Have you done anything different?"

Your client can experience a noticeable decline in visual acuity if critical steps were altered. If the wearing sequence (right lens first or left lens first) or the way the lenses are worn (individually or together) were modified, for example, it can produce immediate blurriness. If certain steps were omitted or added, it can produce the same result. If Step 5 was omitted from the Standard Drill, for example, it can produce slight blurriness.

26.7   CHECK THE EASE OF EXECUTION

Check how the lens is inserted and removed when the patient performs the drill. Is it done smoothly? Is fear minimized during the insertion? During the removal?

26.8   CHECK THE PATIENT'S COMFORT LEVEL

If the patient had never worn contact lenses before, practicing with only the first part of the Preliminary Drill for a week or so can alleviate the discomfort. Initially, the sensitivity to the lens produces excessive tearing, but there should not be any pain. If the patient reports the presence of pain during a follow-up, the cornea may have incurred an abrasion somehow or the lens' edge may be chipped.

Check the integrity of the cornea with a slit lamp. If you do not have one, a magnifying glass and penlight can be effective. Adjust the beam of light at different angles: 30°, 45°, or 60° instead of shining the light directly onto the cornea. Any abrasion would show up clearer. Check the edge of the contact lens with a loupe for signs of chipping. Again, if you do not have a loupe, use a magnifying glass. Check the lens with a radius scope (if you have one) to ensure that the contact lens is not warped.

Excessive discomfort may also be due to the size of the lens. It may be too large. It depends on the gap between the opened lids. You can tell if a lens is too large if it is hard to insert. A diameter of 9.2 mm should fit most patients, but if your patient has a narrow lids opening, reduce the lens' diameter to 9.0 mm.

26.9   CHECK THE WEARING TIME

The patient should remove the lens right after the drill. The wearing time is the duration the lens is on the cornea. By having the lens on too long, the gap between the flange and the cornea allows the tears and contact lens solution to drain and air would eventually seep in. The "draw" would then be over a smaller area due to the reduced meniscus. Eventually, the contact lens would separate from the solution and tears altogether, and the lens would start pushing against the cornea.

The lens would then become an ortho K lens instead of an ortho C lens. Ortho C and ortho K do not mix. One of the warning signs to indicate that the wearing time is too long is that the clarity will decrease prior to removal. Another indication is that objects in the distance are a bit blur after removing the lenses; there is a partial relapse in the improvement gained from the previous attempts, and it takes 5 or 10 min to regain it.

If the patient does not remove the lens after the drill, you have to find out why. Is the patient attempting to combine ortho K with ortho C? Is she engaging in another task at the same time instead of allowing time exclusively for the drill? Is she treating the ortho C lenses as a visual aid?

26.10   CHECK THE FREQUENCY OF WEAR

The frequency of wear refers to how often the patient wears the lenses. If she has mild myopia, it is easy to reset the deviation since the muscles, lens, and eyeball were not severely compromised. The wearing schedule in the short and medium term is less. The goal is to wear them perhaps once every 3 weeks or a month. You want the patient to depend less and less on the lens. She cannot keep resetting the eye neurologically all the time when it is not necessary.

If the patient has high myopia, physiotherapy also needs to be considered. Performing the drills regularly is not just a process of resetting the correct neurological message. The drill also stretches and strengthens the intraocular and extraocular muscles. Although the wearing schedule is more frequent than treating mild or moderate myopia, the lenses are not worn every day just as you would not think of working out in the gym for seven days a week. Similar to the major muscles of your body, the muscles of the eye need rest after a workout.

The frequency of wear is not like ortho K where the patient wears the lenses every night. With ortho C, it is the opposite. Even with severe myopia, the intention is to depend less and less on the lenses. By constantly resetting the neurologically message, the lens and sclera are not given a chance to synchronize.

26.11   CHECK THE RETENTION PERIOD

The wearing schedule's goal is to maintain the improvement and increase the retention period instead of just striving to improve the visual acuity. The latter is a secondary consideration and will take place accordingly. The patient cannot force it.

After performing the drill two times a week for 2 weeks, the retention period should become progressive. To increase the retention period, the client has to wait until the oblique muscles start to tighten up a bit before wearing the lens again and performing the drill. It natural for those muscles to become tight again if you are constantly engaged in near and midrange work.

The retention period should become longer each time the patient performs the drill. You want the client to help you determine the retention period by keeping track of how long it lasts each time she does the drill. At some point, it would peak and that would be the wearing schedule in the interim. (Refer to the chapter *Wearing Schedule* for more information.)

26.12   CHECK THE CONDITION OF THE LENS, PLUNGER, AND CONTACT LENS SOLUTION

If you have a radius scope, check the curvature of the lens. If the lens is slightly warped, the client may be handling it too rough. Check the surface for scratches or scuff marks. Examine the edge for nicks. When storing the lens dry, it can move excessively in the case. Remind the client not to leave them in the car. Even immersed in the solution, the shear force can still chip the edge. Also, the heat can affect the lens. Check the condition of the plunger. If it is losing its suction, replace it. Sometimes, the cup is flattened out when the plunger is collapsed accidentally in the case. The container as well as the plunger should be kept clean. Check the contact lens solution. If it is dirty, remind the client to change it regularly. If it is low, check for leaks. The cap may not sit or screw on properly.

Review contact lens handling and care with the client again. (Refer to the *Addendum* for more information.)

KEYWORDS

- follow-up
- method
- visual acuity test
- resistance

- bad habits
- shock
- experimenting

CHAPTER 27

TROUBLESHOOTING

ABSTRACT

Suppose the patient does not experience the expected outcome; or if he does, suppose there was a relapse. If the problem is not related to any of the items listed in the chapter *Extraneous Variables*, then it may be related to the apparatus or to the method of treatment instead of the eye. In research terminology, the problem probably resides not in the dependent variable but in the independent variable. For example, you may have made a miscalculation in designing the lens, or the patient may have misinterpreted the steps of the drill (assuming that the patient's prescription and K reading are correct). If an adverse factor affecting the design of the lens and/or the application of the drills was dealt with by adhering to protocol, it demonstrates the consistency of applying standardization in seeking a solution.

I also included a case to illustrate that it is actually more difficult to correct a patient with a prescription of −0.25 D in each eye. There is not much room for error and designing the lens can be challenging. One of the stipulations is that you cannot reverse any part of the eye that did not become myopic. The case study alone provides excellent verification on the reliability of ortho C. To avoid the difficulties you may encounter, you may actually want to pass up treating anyone with −0.25 D in both eyes and suggest natural relaxation exercises instead.

27.1 PROBLEM 1: VISUAL ACUITY IMMEDIATELY BECAME BLURRED DUE TO MIXING UP THE LENSES

27.1.1 THE COMPLAINT

A participant with a primary refractive error mentioned that her vision immediately became blurred after she attempted the first step of the Preliminary Drill at home.

27.1.2 THE PROBLEM

An immediate decline in visual acuity after performing Step 1 is a hint that the right and left lenses were switched. It was not her visual acuity prior to ortho C that deteriorated. It was the improved visual acuity she experienced at the clinic after the first application that regressed.

27.1.3 ASSESSMENT

I checked my records, and it indicated that the right lens had a dot. The wearing sequence suggested inserting the right lens in the weaker eye first, and then the left lens in the better eye next. The lab usually places a dot on the right lens to differentiate it from the left lens. The participant confirmed that the right lens has a dot; it was in the contact lens case for the right eye, but she thought she may have reversed the lenses by accident when she was performing the drill. If she switched the lenses, she would have worn the left lens in the weaker right eye first, etc. The degree of blurriness as a result depends on the difference in the flatness of the lens between the right and left eye. If the left lens was a flatter lens, then the blurriness would be more noticeable after Step 1.

27.1.4 PROPOSED SOLUTION

To verify the correct sequence of wear, I asked her to perform Steps 1 and 2 of the Preliminary Drill again. It is the first and second steps that set the tone of the wearing sequence for the rest of the drill. She wore the right lens with the dot first. I then checked her visual acuity afterward.

27.1.5 OUTCOME

Her visual acuity improved after she completed Steps 1 and 2 of the drill. Thus, she had reversed the lenses. I told her to perform the complete drill (Steps 1 to 4) over again to reset her vision.

27.2   PROBLEM 2: VISUAL ACUITY IMMEDIATELY BECAME BLURRED DUE TO ALTERING THE WEARING SEQUENCE

27.2.1   THE COMPLAINT

A participant with a primary refractive error mentioned that her vision immediately became blurred after she attempted the second step of the Preliminary Drill at home.

27.2.2   THE PROBLEM

A decline in visual acuity after performing Step 2 is a hint that the wearing sequence was altered. She already performed the Wearing Sequence Test at the clinic. It was determined that she should wear the right lens first in the weaker right eye and then the left lens next in the better left eye.

27.2.3   ASSESSMENT

I checked if she switched the right and left lenses by accident. Normally, the lab places a dot on lens for the right eye. I found the lenses were stored correctly, but the wearing sequence may have been altered. If she wore the left lens first in the better left eye in Step 1, she would see better at first; but if she proceed to wear the right lens next in the weaker right eye in Step 2, her vision would become worse.

The outcome is different from mixing up the lenses. She did not notice that her vision was blurred until the second step of the Preliminary Drill. If the lenses were switched by accident, her visual acuity would have deteriorated after the first step. (The base curve for each lens was different.)

27.2.4   PROPOSED SOLUTION

To verify the correct wearing sequence, I asked her to perform Steps 1 and 2 of the Preliminary Drill again by wear the right lens first.

27.2.5   OUTCOME

Her visual acuity improved after she completed the Wearing Sequence Test.

27.2.6   DISCUSSION

Suppose she just started the procedure at your clinic, and there was no improvement in visual acuity after the lenses were worn in the correct order. There is the possibility that the suggested sequence according to the visual acuity test (and prescription) is incorrect. To verify the change in wearing sequence, take out the left lens that was inserted last in the left eye and insert the right lens in the right eye again. If after wearing the right lens and performing the Distance Drill produces better results, then you know the supposedly weaker right eye improved at a quicker rate than the better eye. (Refer to the chapter *The Procedure* for more information.)

The above scenario would also suggest the possibility that her Add (or presbyopia) is higher than the Sphere. Check her prescription to verify that there is nothing in the Add portion. If there is a measurement for her add, make sure that it is not higher than her sphere. If it is higher, you may have a scenario where you would have to treat her presbyopia instead of myopia. It involves a different wearing sequence.

If her prescription was OD −0.75 D, OS −0.50 D, and Add +1.75 D, you have to treat her presbyopia to correct her myopia. I cannot go into the treatment here. It involves a different methodology. It is not just a matter of reversing the wearing sequence.

27.3   PROBLEM 3: VISUAL ACUITY BECAME BLURRED AFTER 1 DAY

27.3.1   THE COMPLAINT

A participant mentioned that his vision became blurred the next day after he attempted the Preliminary Drill. It was more noticeable during the evening. He has anisometropia.

27.3.2 THE PROBLEM

When the visual acuity becomes blurred after 1 day, most likely the crystalline lens or eyeball was overcorrected. According to protocol, you cannot overcorrect any part of the eye beyond how much it deviated. The symptom did not occur immediately. If it took longer to set in, such as after 1 h or after 1 day, the crystalline lens or eyeball was not overcorrected by much; but it was still overcorrected.

27.3.3 ASSESSMENT

He confirmed that the wearing sequence was correct, and he performed Steps 1 and 2 within the allotted time. He performs the drill mostly on a slightly cloudy day or on a clear day without any glare interfering with the drill. There was no change in his working habits in front of the computer. He continues to try to maintain the correct distance, and he followed the 20/20 rule. I watched how he performed the Preliminary Drill at the clinic. He occluded one eye in Steps 1 and 2 instead of leaving them uncovered. By covering one eye, it exposed the lens' occluded neutral shape. It is a slightly more myopic shape. The drill then becomes a different drill (which I did not cover in this publication). It is a more intense drill. The overcorrection produced a deterioration.

27.3.4 PROPOSED SOLUTION

Perform the preliminary drill without covering the eye in Steps 1 and 2.

27.3.5 OUTCOME

His visual acuity was better after he performed the Preliminary Drill without occluding the other eye in Steps 1 and 2.

27.4 PROBLEM 4: RETENTION PERIOD GRADUALLY REGRESSED AFTER REACHING ITS PEAK

27.4.1 THE COMPLAINT

A participant initially performed the Preliminary Drill to treat anisome-tropia. She reached the phase in the wearing schedule where her visual acuity remained clear for a month without performing any drill. She performs the drill once a month for maintenance. Lately, the retention period regressed. Her vision started to become blur after 1 week to indicate that she had to perform the drill again, and the blurriness was not as subtle. (The deterioration, however, did not completely regress back to the original myopic state prior to her treatment.)

Her visual acuity tests were as follows:

Visual acuity of naked eye:
Both: Line 6
Right: Line 5
Left: Line 6

Former visual acuity of naked eye at its peak after ortho C:
Both: Line 9 − 2
Right: Line 8
Left: Line 8 − 3

Original visual acuity of naked eye prior to ortho C:
Both: Line 5 − 2
Right: Line 3
Left: Line 4 − 1

27.4.2   THE PROBLEM

If the retention lasted only a week when its duration used to be a month, a resistance had built up. Although she gained maximum improvement, the Preliminary Drill was not sufficient to insulate it against frequent exposure to normal day-to-day work and to different forms of instrument myopia. I told her that she eventually had to switch to the Modified Preliminary Drill. She went on vacation and delayed the transition to the new drill.

27.4.3   ASSESSMENT

I checked how the participant did the drill. She performed the steps correctly and the wearing sequence was correct. She reported that there was no change in her working habits in front of the computer. She continues to try to maintain the correct distance, and she followed the 20/20 rule. Thus, she was not constantly exposed to near-point stress.

27.4.4 PROPOSED SOLUTION

I switched her over to the Modified Preliminary Drill.

27.4.5 OUTCOME

Her binocular visual acuity improved by three lines on the Snellen chart after she performed the Modified Preliminary Drill. It prolonged the retention period. She also reported that she sees clearer at night.

27.5 PROBLEM 5: DISPROPORTIONATE V/A READING AFTER SWITCHING OVER TO THE MODIFIED PRELIMINARY DRILL

27.5.1 THE PROBLEM

A patient experienced a disproportionate improvement in visual acuity after performing the Modified Preliminary Drill. Her weaker eye improved more than her better eye. It persisted for 2 weeks after performing the drill just once.

In addition to anisometropia, there was a trace of anisometropic amblyopia. If she covered her better eye without leaving a gap, the weaker eye would deteriorate by as much as three lines on the Snellen chart. By leaving a gap between the better eye and the occluder, the weaker eye sees better; the wider the gap, the better the weaker eye's visual acuity. If she covered the eye completely when performing the drill, especially the Snellen chart part of the drill, her visual acuity would become blurred. She needs to leave a gap between her eye and the palm of her hand.

> *Rx prior to ortho C*:
> Right −2.00
> Left −1.00
>
> *Visual acuity after performing the preliminary drill*:
> Both: Line 8
> Right: Line 8
> Left: Line 7

27.5.2   ASSESSMENT

I initially instructed the participant to start with the right eye when performing the Preliminary Drill. It was the weaker eye. She was supposed to start with the left better eye after switching over to the Modified Preliminary Drill to address anisometropic amblyopia, but she continued with the previous wearing sequence. The outcome was that the weaker eye improved more. The neuropathway is different in compound anisometropia and anisometropic amblyopia.

27.5.3   PROPOSED SOLUTION

I had the participant perform the Modified Preliminary Drill starting with the left eye instead of the right.

27.5.4   OUTCOME

Her improved visual acuity became proportionate after she performed the Modified Preliminary Drill starting with the left better eye. The retention period increased. She also reported that she sees clearer at night while driving.

> *Her visual acuity was as follows*:
> Both: Line 9 (read it from left to right)
> Right: Line 8
> Left: Line 9 (reading it backwards from right to left)

27.5.5   DISCUSSION

Starting with the left eye, or the better eye, is contrary to the conventional wearing sequence. The participant followed the regular sequence when she performed the Preliminary Drill. She started with the right weaker eye first. However, it did not conform to the Modified Preliminary Drill. It does not mean the weaker eye is more receptive to the drill. The neuropathway is different. It seemed that the Modified Preliminary Drill strives to reestablish how the anisometropic amblyopic eye should function. Normally, the binocular vision of the myopic eye takes on the visual acuity of the better eye, but the anisometropic eye often sees clearer with the better eye compared with both eyes.

In this particular case, her binocular vision is equal to her left eye. It is an indication that the weaker eye released its influence over the better eye. A hint that neurology contributed to the difficulty was that she was able to read line 9 normally with both eyes from left to right, but she could only read line 9 backwards with the left eye from right to left.

27.6   PROBLEM 6: NO IMPROVEMENT IN VISUAL ACUITY AFTER CONDUCTING THE FIRST RESISTANCE TEST

27.6.1   THE COMPLAINT

The participant was in his 30s, and his prescription was OD −1.75 and OS −1.75. He came from Australia to visit me to ensure that he performs the procedure correctly. I expected good results because he told me that he never wore his glasses—even when he drives.

After he performed the first resistance test, he mentioned that the Snellen test card does not look any different:

> *Visual acuity of naked eye prior to any drills*:
> Both: Line 4
> *Visual acuity after first resistance test*:
> Both: Line 4

27.6.2   THE PROBLEM

He told me that he had worn contact lenses only about half a dozen times over the year, but it may be enough to induce a partial spasm. He also never wore his glasses—even when he drives. For short distances, it might be okay, but driving for long periods can produce an excessive "effort to see" since he can only see down to line 4 on the eye chart.

27.6.3   ASSESSMENT

The first part of the Preliminary Drill (Steps 1 and 2) is equivalent to the first resistance test. It measures the flexibility of the ciliary muscle. It is more susceptible to near-point stress than the rectus muscles. If there is no improvement in visual acuity after the patient performs the first resistance test, it is an indication that the ciliary muscle is tense. It does not always mean, however, that spasticity has set in. He may just have a partial resistance. I had to determine the degree of resistance.

27.6.4 PROPOSED SOLUTION

I told him to continue with the second part of the Preliminary Drill (Steps 3 and 4) which is actually equivalent to the second resistance test. It can still nudge a partial improvement despite a lack in response to the first resistance test. The resistance tests do not just map out the degree of resistance. Each test also presents different conditions to activate the ciliary muscle to relax.

Sometimes, the Snellen Chart Drill (which is the drill involved in the second resistance test) will bring better results if the ciliary muscle was not that tense. If too much time had lapsed from the first resistance test, he would have to perform the Preliminary Drill again starting from Step 1; but since I took the visual acuity test quickly after the first resistance test, I assumed that the ciliary muscle was still sufficiently relaxed.

27.6.5 OUTCOME

A partial improvement did not register after he completed Step 3 of the Preliminary Drill, but he could see down to line 7 on the Snellen chart after he performed Step 4. Although there was a three-line improvement, it is still considered a partial improvement. He could see down to line 7 on the test card, but the blurriness started at line 4. Line 7 was somewhat blur, but he could still see it. Although the stress was directly induced by wearing contact lenses, the tension was not that great. He only wore them for about half a dozen times over the year.

It is also possible for someone with a low resistance to gain a three-line improvement down to line 7, but the difference is that the blurriness would usually start at line 7 or line 6. An eye with a partial resistance to ortho C tends to experience a higher degree of blurriness—but not uniform blurriness as experienced by someone with a loss of depth perception.

27.6.6 DISCUSSION

He may eventually have to perform the Standard Drill or Modified Preliminary Drill. Just as in the case of treating anisometropia, it may be too unstable to continuing performing the Preliminary Drill since it mainly addresses the crystalline lens. It is possible for a resistance to build up.

27.7   PROBLEM 7: NO IMPROVEMENT IN VISUAL ACUITY AFTER CONDUCTING THE FIRST, SECOND, AND THIRD RESISTANCE TEST

27.7.1   THE COMPLAINT

The patient was 15 years of age. Her prescription was OD −1.00 D and OS −1.00 D. The first, second, and third resistance test did not produce any improvement in visual acuity. Her partial resistance was very high. There was only a partial response to the fourth resistance test. Her visual acuity tests were as follows:

> *Visual acuity of naked eye prior to any drills*:
> Both: Line 3
> Right: Line 2
> Left: Line 2
> *Visual acuity after the fourth resistance tests*:
> Both: Line 5

27.7.2   THE PROBLEM

There is the possibility that her myopia started during development. Her myopia set in only a couple of years ago. Considering her age, developmental factors may interfere with ortho C. If the crystalline lens did not bulged sufficiently in response to near-point stress, then the eyeball inherited most of the deformation. There were no other extraneous variables that may cause the ciliary muscle to spasm. She never wore glasses to read or to work in front of the computer. She maintained the proper distance for the near and midrange.

27.7.3   ASSESSMENT

Her visual acuity with the naked eye attested to the loss in depth perception. Under normal conditions with adequate lighting prior to ortho C, she only read down to line 3. The chart was uniformly blurred. It hinted that most of the deviation resided in the eyeball. A −1.00 D eye should see much better. Even without the assistance of the crystalline lens, she should see down to line 4 or the 20/50 line. Thus, although the tension was indirectly induced, the crystalline lens did not assume the proper myopic shape. The eyeball elongated more than usual. (Refer to the *Addendum* for more information.)

27.7.4   PROPOSED SOLUTION

Her prescription was actually closer to −1.50 D. She sees down to line 3 (just barely). To activate the eye to "shift," the flatness factor needs to be higher than 1.0 D. I fitted her with a flatness factor of 1.50 D. The intention of a flatter lens is to stimulate the eyeball to "shift." I had her perform the Modified Standard Drill. (Later she would attempt the Modified Preliminary Drill.)

27.7.5   OUTCOME

Her binocular visual acuity improved by another line (to line 6) after applying the Modified Standard Drill.

27.8   PROBLEM 8: MILD MYOPIA BECAME WORSE AFTER THE WEARING SEQUENCE TEST

27.8.1   THE COMPLAINT

The participant had laser surgery last year. He noticed that his vision was starting to regress and wanted to try ortho C instead of having a "touch up" (by reapplying the laser to the cornea). His prescription was OD −0.25 D and OS −0.25 D. Although the prescription is the same in each eye, there is a difference in visual acuity of one line on the Snellen chart.

27.8.2   THE PROBLEM

A prescription of OD −0.25 D and OS −0.25 D can be difficult to correct. The deviation is slight and leaves little room for error. Although his prescription before laser surgery was −3.00 D, a lens 0.25 D flatter than mid K can still be too flat. I am treating his existing prescription—not his previous prescription. A difference in visual acuity of one line on the Snellen chart can pose a problem.

27.8.3 ASSESSMENT

I mentioned earlier that you should pass up on attempting to treat such a prescription. There is hardly any room for error. The following case is for information only to illustrate the complications that you may encounter.

27.8.4 ATTEMPTED TREATMENT

After I received the lens from the lab, I conducted a visual acuity test first for the distance without any visual aid:

> Both: Line 9 − 1
> Right: Line 7 + 5
> Left: Line 8 + 5

The assumption was that his right eye is the weaker eye. A Wearing Sequence Test was conducted as follows:

1. After inserting a lens with a flatness of 0.25 D on the right eye, the results were as follows:
    Both: Line 10
    Right: Line 8 + 4
    Left: Line 7
    The left eye lost 1.5 lines due to the indirect effect.

2. After inserting a lens with a flatness of 0.25 D on the left eye, the results were as follows:
    Both: Line 8 + 5
    Right: Line 8
    Left: Line 8 − 2 + 5

    The left eye almost gained the visual acuity lost in Step 1, but the right eye lost about half a line compared to Step 1. His binocular vision lost about 1.5 lines compared to Step 1. At first, I thought it was due to an incorrect sequence.

3. After inserting a lens with a flatness of 0.25 D on the right eye again, the results were as follows:

    Both: Line 8

    His binocular vision lost about half a line compared to Step 2 and two lines compared to Step 1. He mentioned that line 8 was blurry. The purpose of wearing the lens in the right eye again was to test if the wearing sequence was reversed. If the left eye happens to be the weaker eye instead of the right, then the proper wearing sequence should be left eye first and then the right. By just inserting the lens in the right eye again, it would verify that possibility (as discussed in the earlier problem on altering the wearing sequence). But further deterioration in his binocular vision as a result suggested that the original assumption was correct—that the right eye was the weaker eye. It also suggested that the decline in visual acuity in Step 2 was due to a lens that was too flat.

4. After inserting a lens with a flatness of 0.25 D on the left eye again, the results were as follows:
    Both: Line 8
    He mentioned that line 8 looked better, and he could also read some of line 9.

Since Step 3 indicated that the wearing sequence was not reversed, I had to complete Step 4 to reset his vision. Otherwise he would continue to see worse. After he did the distance drill with the lens in the left eye, his vision was starting to recover. The partial recovery after wearing the left lens again in Step 4 confirmed that the initial wear sequence of right eye first and then left was correct. The blurriness in v/a was not due to an improper wearing sequence but to the lenses' flatness factor.

27.8.5 PROPOSED SOLUTION

I redesigned the lenses. The flatness factor for the better eye would be on the steep K, and the lens' flatness for the weaker eye would be 0.25 D flatter than steep K. There was a difference in visual acuity of one line on the Snellen chart. The flatness factor for the better eye is on steep K to eliminate the risk that a direct influence would overcorrect the eye if it was on the mid K. The lens' flatness for the weaker eye is 0.25 D flatter than steep K because the margin of error is not as restrictive as the other eye. A flatter lens on the weaker eye did not overcorrect the crystalline lens of the better eye. The indirect effect did not produce a tear layer.

27.8.6 OUTCOME

After performing the Standard Drill with the above lenses starting with the left eye first (the better eye), the results were as follows:
Both: Line 9 + 5
Right: Line 9
Left: Line 9

27.8.7 DISCUSSION

His original prescription was −3.00 D before he had laser surgery. His prescription OD −0.25 D and OS −0.25 D did not offer much leeway for a "focal point draw." The laser surgery already compensated the previous deviation in the lens and eyeball. By designing a pair of lenses OD 0.25 D and OS 0.25 D flatter than mid K, it induced an overcorrection. It demonstrates that ortho C cannot force the crystalline lens or eyeball to reverse beyond the residual deviation of −0.25 D—as mentioned in the chapter *Reinstating the Correct Message*.

KEYWORDS

- Preliminary Drill
- Modified Preliminary Drill
- Modified Standard Drill
- visual acuity test
- wearing sequence test
- first resistance test
- second resistance test

CHAPTER 28

CASE EXAMPLES

ABSTRACT

The verification of the selected case examples are based on a pretest–posttest design. The main criticism of a pretest–posttest design from a research point of view is the lack of internal and external validity because I am just measuring one group instead of two as exemplified in the chapter *Reinstating the Correct Message*. But I am not just depending on the outcomes of the pretests and posttests of the experimental groups alone. I am also comparing them to archival data. The results are identical to researched outcomes conducted with other participants over the years. It is similar to hundreds of other cases where I adopted the same method and specifications to treat primary and secondary refractive errors. The outcomes demonstrate the consistency of applying standardization in treating a specific problem.

The following are examples of actual cases where I applied the recommended drill (the method) and flatness factor (the specifications of the contact lens) to treat a specific primary or secondary refractive error: mild myopia, moderate myopia, high astigmatism, compound anisometropia and anisometropic amblyopia, and compound anisometropia and high astigmatism.

28.1 CASE 1: MILD MYOPIA

Joe had mild myopia. The prescription of each eye was −0.50 D.

28.1.1 RX

Right eye: −0.50 D
Left eye: −0.50 D

28.1.2   KERATOMETER READING

I took Joe's keratometer reading (K reading):

> Right: 43.50 @ 180/44.50 @ 90
> Left: 43.75 @ 180/44.50 @ 90

> I then calculated the mid K.

28.1.3   MID K:

> Right: 44.00 D
> Left: 44.12 D

> From the mid K, I calculated the base curve.

28.1.4   BASE CURVE

> Right: 44.00 D − 0.50 D = 43.50 D = 7.76 mm
> Left: 44.12 D − 0.50 D = 43.62 D = 7.74 mm

28.1.5   ASSESSMENT

I conducted a visual acuity test to determine which eye was the weaker eye. The information was not obvious from the written prescription. From the following v/a test, I predicted that the left eye was the weaker eye. Each eye started to see a bit blur one line before the best line he could read (line 8) instead of two or three lines before it. Thus, his vertical depth perception was normal.

> *v/a of naked eye:*
> Both: Line 8 + 4
> Right: Line 8 − 2 (chart starts to blur at line 7)
> Left: Line 7 (chart starts to blur at line 6)

28.1.6   THE TREATMENT

After I received the lenses, I took another visual acuity test. I wanted to know how the participant sees on that day. From the following v/a test, his binocular vision was a bit worse compared to the initial visit, but his monocular vision was essentially the same. The new benchmark established a new set of before and after results. It also ensured that he was not subjected to any negative factors since the last time we met that may displace the eye outside the myopic model. I intended to apply the modified preliminary drill.

> *v/a before performing any drill*:
> Both: Line 8
> Right: Line 8 − 2
> Left: Line 7

He was very sensitive to having something on his cornea. I omitted the Wearing Sequence Test to reduce the number of times he needs to insert and remove the lens. I had him start with the left eye first. From the v/a test, it was his weaker eye. The results of the Modified Preliminary Drill were as follows:

> *v/a after performing the Modified Preliminary Drill*:
> Both: Line 10
> Right: Line 10
> Left: Line 9 −2

28.1.7   FOLLOW-UP

I asked him to return after 2 weeks for a follow-up to check his retention. He did not perform the drill during that period. He was still very sensitive to the lenses. His visual acuity was as follows:

> *v/a 2 weeks later*:
> Both: Line 10 − 3
> Right: Line 9 − 2
> Left: Line 9 − 3

Since he maintained most of the improvement, it confirmed his receptiveness to ortho C. It is an example of an eye with a low resistance to ortho C: when there was an immediate improvement after the Modified Preliminary Drill and when the improvement was maintained for 2 weeks after the first application. He performed the drill again to increase the retention period. I had him return after 2 weeks. His visual acuity was as follows:

> *v/a 2 weeks later:*
> Both: Line 11
> Right: Line 10 − 4
> Left: Line 10 − 3

His visual acuity was better than the last follow-up. It is suggested that the retention could have lasted longer before he had to perform the drill again. I told him to check the v/a daily to determine the new retention period.

28.2   CASE 2: MODERATE MYOPIA

Tonya had moderate myopia. The prescription of each eye was

28.2.1   RX

> Right eye: −1.00
> Left eye: −1.00

28.2.2   K READING

I took Tonya's keratometer reading:
> Right: 40.50 @ 180/41.50 @ 90
> Left: 40.00 @ 180/41.50 @ 90

28.2.3   MID K:

> Right: 41.00 D
> Left: 40.75 D

From the mid K, I calculated the base curve.

28.2.4   BASE CURVE:

Right: $41.00 \text{ D} - 1.00 \text{ D} = 40.00 \text{ D} = 8.44 \text{ mm}$
Left: $40.75 \text{ D} - 1.00 \text{ D} = 39.75 \text{ D} = 8.49 \text{ mm}$

28.2.5   ASSESSMENT

I conducted a visual acuity test to determine which eye was the weaker eye. The information was not obvious from the written prescription. From the following v/a test, each eye can see down to line 5, but she mentioned that the left eye sees a bit better when looking at the chart as a whole. Each eye started to see a bit blur at the best line she could read instead of two or three lines before it. Thus, her vertical depth perception was normal.

v/a of naked eye:
Both: Line 7
Right: Line 5
Left: Line 5

28.2.6   THE TREATMENT

After I received the lenses, I took another visual acuity test. I wanted to know how she sees on that day. From the following v/a test, it was the same as the week before.

v/a before performing any drill:
Both: Line 7
Right: Line 5
Left: Line 5

It was the first time she wore contact lenses, and she was very apprehensive. I decided that she start with the Wearing Sequence Test. It is equivalent to the first part of the Preliminary Drill. The plan was to have her try just the first part of the Preliminary Drill first to ease her into adapting to the contact lens. She was unable to insert the lens herself. I had to insert it for her.

She continued to resist keeping her eyes open. When I did manage to insert the right lens, she performed the Distant Drill. The result was as follows:

> *v/a after performing Step 1 of the Wearing Sequence Test*:
> Both: Line 8 − 1

It was also a struggle inserting the left lens. When I managed to insert it, she performed the Distance Drill. The improvement in visual acuity confirmed that the wearing sequence is correct. The result was as follows:

> *v/a after performing Step 2 of the Wearing Sequence Test*:
> Both: Line 8 + 5

It was difficult to insert the right lens back on to continue with the Preliminary Drill. I stopped after applying the Wearing Sequence Test which was equivalent to the first part of the Preliminary Drill. I decided to order a lens with a smaller diameter. I reduced the diameter of the lens from 9.2 to 9.0 mm.

28.2.7   FOLLOW-UP

I asked her return after 2 weeks for a follow-up. Her visual acuity after that period was as follows:

v/a 2 weeks later:
Both: Line 8 − 4
Right: Line 7 − 1
Left: Line 7 − 1

There was a slight fluctuation in her binocular vision which was to be expected after applying just the first part of the Preliminary Drill. The crystalline lens performed all the work in bringing a distant object into focus. It compensated for its own myopic shape as well as the myopic shape of the eyeball. The increase in "effort to see" produced a slight regression.

28.2.8   APPLYING THE STANDARD DRILL

The new lenses fitted better. Although there was still tearing, they were not as uncomfortable as the previous pair. The results of performing the Standard Drill were as follows:

> *v/a after performing the Standard Drill*:
> Both: $10 - 2$
> Rright: $8 - 4 + 5$
> Left: $8 - 1 + 3$

28.3   CASE 3: HIGH ASTIGMATISM

Doug had compound astigmatism. He was one of my international participants who I treated online. I had sent to him instructions on contact lens insertion and removal, information on how to apply a plunger (contact lens remover), and preliminary information on contact lens handling and care. (Refer to the *Addendum* on these topics.)

His prescription was as follows:

28.3.1   RX

> Right eye: $-1.50 - 1.25 \times 180$
> Left eye: $-1.50 - 1.25 \times 180$

I took into account the high astigmatism while calculating the lens' flatness factor. From the Flatness Factor chart, the flatness of the lens is 1.75 D. I subtracted 1.75 D from mid K to arrive at the base curve as in the calculation below.

28.3.2   K READING

Doug's keratometer reading was as follows:

> Right eye: 44.00 @ 180/46.50 @ 90
> Left eye: 44.00 @ 180/46.50 @ 90

I then calculated the mid K based on the specifications for compound astigmatism:

28.3.3 MID K:

Right: $44.00 + 46.50/2 = 45.25$
Left: $44.00 + 46.50/2 = 45.25$

From the mid K, I calculated the base curve:

28.3.4 BASE CURVE:

Right eye: $45.25 - 1.75 = 43.50 = 7.75$
Left eye: $45.25 - 1.75 = 43.50 = 7.75$

The K reading for both eyes are the same. I designed both lenses with the same base curve. The lenses I gave were as follows:

28.3.5 LENSES GIVEN

Right eye: 7.75 mm
Left eye: 7.75 mm

28.3.6 ASSESSMENT

I asked Doug to conduct a Visual Acuity Test to determine which eye is the weaker eye. I needed that information before introducing any drills. In good lighting (by a source of natural light outside), his visual acuity was as follows:

v/a of naked eye:
Both: Line 3 + 2
Right: Line 2
Left: Line 3

v/a with −0.50 D glasses:
Both: Line 7
Right: Line 5
Left: Line 6

28.3.7   THE TREATMENT

I suggested that he perform the First Resistance Test because his astigmatism was just over −1.00 D. The First Resistance Test is equivalent to the first part of the Preliminary Drill. Compound astigmatism with high astigmatism usually does not respond well to the First Resistance Test. According to the v/a test, his weaker eye is the right eye. He performed Step 1 of the First Resistance Test with just the right lens on. Both eyes were kept opened while he performed the Distance Drill. Then he performed Step 2 with just the left lens on. Both eyes were kept opened while he performed the Distance Drill.

v/a of naked eye before performing the First Resistance Test:
Both: Line 4
Right: Line 2
Left: Line 3

v/a with −0.50 D glasses before performing the First Resistance Test:
Both: Line 6
Right: Line 4
Left: Line 5

v/a of naked eye after performing the First Resistance Test:
Both: Line 4
Right: Line 2
Left: Line 4

v/a with −0.50 D glasses after performing the First Resistance Test:
Both: Line 6
Right: Line 3 + 2
Left: Line 5 + 3

As expected there was not much change in his visual acuity. It does not mean that he is not a good candidate for ortho C. The resistance test indicated that there was a partial resistance. It was probably due to his high astigmatism. Unlike the type of partial resistance where the eye deviated from the myopic model, it can be resolved by performing the Modified Preliminary Drill.

The results of the Modified Preliminary Drill were as follows:

> *v/a of naked eye after performing the Modified Preliminary Drill*:
> Both: Line 10
> Right: Line 9
> Left: Line 9 + 6

28.3.8 DISCUSSION

The resistance test suggested that he was not a good candidate for the Standard Drill. The secondary refractive error, his compound myopia and astigmatism, took precedence. Sometimes performing just the first part of the Standard Drill gives excellent results. The first part of the drill is slightly more intense than the Modified Preliminary Drill due to the multiplier effect. The results may last for weeks, but when the patient attempts the drill again, it is possible to experience a relapse due to an overcorrection. The Modified Preliminary Drill, on the other hand, attends to the lens and eyeball in the right proportion.

28.4 CASE 4: ANISOMETROPIA

Jane had anisometropia. The disparity in prescription between the right and left eye is −1.00 D. The right eye is in the midrange, and the left eye is in the moderately myopic.

28.4.1 RX

> Right eye: −2.00 D
> Left eye: −1.00 D

28.4.2   K READING

I also took Jane's keratometer reading as follows:

> Right: 42.25 @ 180/43.25 @ 90
> Left: 42.25 @ 180/43.25 @ 90
> I then calculated the mid K.

28.4.3   MID K:

> Right: 42.75 D
> Left: 42.75 D
> From the mid K, I calculated the base curve.

28.4.4   BASE CURVE:

> Right: 42.75 D − 2.00 D = 40.75 D = 8.28 mm
> Left: 42.75 D − 2.00 D = 40.75 D = 8.28 mm

28.4.5   ASSESSMENT

I checked her visual acuity. There was the presence of anisometropic amblyopia. There were wide swings in visual acuity when she covered the better eye completely compared to leaving a gap between the better eye and the occluder. She was sensitive to instrument myopia.

From her prescription, the right eye is the weaker eye. From the following v/a test, there was a disparity of one line between the right and left eye.

> *v/a of naked eye*:
> Both: Line 5 − 2
> Right: Line 3
> Left: Line 4 − 1

28.4.6   THE TREATMENT

I made the lenses 2.00 D flatter than mid K. It is the standard flatness if the weaker eye has midrange myopia (from −2.00 D to −2.75 D). After I received the lenses, I took another visual acuity test. I want to check that the pretest was the same. From the following v/a test, it was almost similar to her initial visit.

> *v/a of naked eye before performing the Preliminary Drill*:
> Both: Line 5 − 2
> Right: Line 3
> Left: Line 4

I had her perform the Preliminary Drill. I can tell from the v/a test that the weaker eye was the right eye. The wearing sequence was the right lens first and then the left. I quickly took a v/a test after Steps 1 and 2 (which is equivalent to the First Resistance Test). I want to perform a resistance test at the same time.

> *v/a of naked eye after performing Steps 1 and 2 of the Preliminary Drill*:
> Both: Line 8

She was responsive to the First Resistance Test. (The First Resistance Test is equal to Steps 1 and 2 of the Preliminary Drill.) She then continued with Second Resistance Test. (The Second Resistance Test is equal to Steps 3 and 4 of the Preliminary Drill.) The wearing sequence is the same as the first part of the drill. I quickly took a v/a test after Steps 3 and 4.

> *v/a of naked eye after performing Steps 3 and 4 of the Preliminary Drill*:
> Both: Line 9
> Right: Line 7
> Left: Line 9 + 6

28.4.7   DISCUSSION

It is not unusual for an anisometropic amblyopic participant to have the better eye improve more than what she sees with both eyes. It is the opposite outcome of a participant with myopia. After a few weeks, her anisometropic amblyopia put up a resistance to the Preliminary Drill. I eventually had to apply the Modified Preliminary Drill to prolong the retention period. She had to perform the drill consistently, about once a week, at first. After about a month, the retention period increased to 2 weeks. She then did the drill once every 2 weeks for about another 2 months. At the time I was making the entry, the retention period increased to about 3 weeks. She experienced clearer vision at night.

28.5   CASE 5: ANISOMETROPIA AND ASTIGMATISM

The participant had anisometropia, anisometropic amblyopia, and high astigmatism. She claims that her astigmatism was induced by brain trauma injury (BTI). She was a skater. She fell and landed hard on her forehead during a national competition when a competitor bumped into her. Although she had mild myopia prior to her BTI, she found that her vision was worse after the BTI. She experienced vertical heterophoria, loss of certain parts in her field of vision, frequent headaches, feeling nauseous sometimes while driving (when coming along a row of trees for instance), pupils not reacting to light changes, and double vision.

The following was her autorefraction reading. An autorefraction reading, which is an objective exam, was taken instead of a conventional subjective eye exam. After a month, she still sees worse in a subjective eye exam due to her BTI, and she could not wear the glasses based on those measurements. She was wondering if my method could improve her visual acuity.

Her initial autorefraction reading was as follows:

OD: $-0.75 - 0.75 \times 124$ and OS: $-1.50 - 1.00 \times 71$
v/a of naked eye:
Both: Line 4 + 2
Right: Line 3 + 2
Left: Line 3 − 1

28.5.1   ASSESSMENT

Her autorefractive reading indicates that she has high astigmatism. She told me she did not have any astigmatism before the accident. A mild myopic eye is more sensitive to astigmatism. In this case, the amount of astigmatism is equivalent to 100% of the sphere in the right eye. I checked her for anisometropic amblyopia, and it was present in her left eye. Her high astigmatism in conjunction with anisometropia and anisometropic amblyopia could contribute to her double vision. If the astigmatism was neurologically induced by TBI, perhaps it could be removed just as readily by resetting the correct neurological message.

28.5.2   THE TREATMENT

I intended to apply the Modified Preliminary Drill. It was designed to treat compound astigmatism. Since I am targeting her astigmatism, it was not necessary to have her perform the Preliminary Drill first to attend to her anisometropia.

28.5.3   OUTCOME

After applying the Modified Preliminary Drill for a couple of times, she had a lower autorefraction reading as follows:

> OD $-0.25 - 1.00 \times 127$ and OS $-1.00 - 1.00 \times 72$
> Her visual acuity improved as follows:
> Both: 8 + 4
> Right: 7 + 4
> Left: 4 + 1

28.5.4   DISCUSSION

An autorefraction measurement is mainly attributed to the eyeball. It is an objective exam. It bypasses the lens since the subject does not have an input. The crystalline lens does not participate in the measurement. It assumes a neutral shape.

The Modified Preliminary Drill was able to reduce the elongation of the myopic eyeball. The cylinder remained unchanged. The compensation does not show up when the lens is in a neutral shape during the autorefraction reading. It compensates for the astigmatism when there is a "focal point draw" as indicated by her binocular vision in the visual acuity test when the crystalline lens was allowed to take part.

According to her K reading, her corneal astigmatism was about −1.00 D. The Modified Preliminary Drill was able to mask it. Otherwise there was no way she was able to read about half of line 9 if the astigmatism was present. Any physical improvement of the corneal distortion itself would be a long-term endeavor as mentioned in the chapter *Treating Astigmatism*.

The left eye continued to offer a high resistance. It was probably due to the BTI. It induced astigmatism along with anisometropia and anisome-tropic amblyopia. If it was not for the induced astigmatism, the disparity between the right and left eye would have been reduced significantly. But it can be resolved by the application of monovision. (Refer to the chapter *Treating Anisometropia* for more information on monovision.)

KEYWORDS

- mild myopia
- moderate myopia
- astigmatism
- anisometropia
- anisometropic amblyopia
- autorefraction
- keratometer reading

CHAPTER 29

SPECIFICATIONS: FEATURES OF AN ORTHO C LENS

ABSTRACT

The specifications are given for a contact lens' flatness in reference to the different disparities and ranges for myopia, anisometropia, and compound anisometropia and astigmatism. Its flatness is also given for the different ranges of astigmatism in the compound myopic and astigmatic eye. A conversion chart from diopters to millimeters of radius is also given. The conversion to millimeters of radius must be made before you can order online or from a lab.

An ortho C lens has the following features:

- There is no prescription. It is a plain contact lens.
- The thickness is 0.15 mm.
- The diameter is 9.2 mm (or 9.0 mm in special cases with narrow lids opening).
- The material should be Boston EO or equivalent (such as Fluoroperm 60).
- The lens' flatness for mild or moderate myopia depends on the disparity in prescription between the right and left eye. Refer to the specifications below for the "flatness factor" for mild and moderate myopia.
- The lens' flatness for compound astigmatism depends on the degree of astigmatism. Refer to the specifications below for the "flatness factor" for mild and moderate myopia and varying degrees of astigmatism.

29.1   FLATNESS FACTOR

The following provides the recommended drills and flatness for a "plano" contact lens (a lens with no prescription) in relation to mild or moderate myopia with different disparities between the right and left eye.

29.1.1   MILD AND MODERATE MYOPIA

29.1.1.1   NO DISPARITY

• For example, OD −1.00 D, OS −1.00 D

If there is no difference in the mild or moderate prescription between the right and left eye, the flatness factor for the right and left lens is equal to the absolute value of the prescription for the right and left eye. In the above example, the flatness factor would be OD 1.00 D and OS 1.00 D flatter than the curvature of the cornea determined at mid K.

Type of drill: Standard Drill.

29.1.1.2   DISPARITY OF −0.25 D

• For example, OD −1.25 D, OS −1.50 D

If the difference in the mild or moderate prescription between the right and left eye is −0.25, the flatness factor for the right and left lens is equal to the absolute value of the prescription for the right and left eye. In the above example, the flatness factor would be OD 1.25 D and OS 1.50 D flatter than the curvature of the cornea determined at mid K.

Type of drill: Standard Drill.

29.1.1.3   DISPARITY OF −0.50 D

• For example, OD −1.25 D, OS −1.75 D

If the difference in the mild or moderate prescription between the right and left eye is −0.50, the flatness factor for the better eye is equal to the absolute value of its prescription plus 0.25 D. The lens' flatness for the weaker eye is equal to the absolute value of its prescription less 0.25 D. In the above example, the flatness factor would be OD 1.50 D and OS 1.50 D flatter than the curvature of the cornea determined at mid K.

Type of drill: Modified Preliminary Drill.

29.1.1.4 DISPARITY OF –0.75 D

- For example, OD –1.00 D, OD –1.75 D

If the difference in the mild or moderate prescription between the right and left eye is −0.75, the flatness factor for the right and left lens is equal to the absolute value of the weaker eye. In the above example, the flatness factor would be OD 1.75 and OS 1.75 flatter than the curvature of the cornea determined at mid K. The maximum flatness would be 2.0 D if the weaker eye is in the midrange. If the patient's prescription is OD −1.50 D and OS −2.25 D, for example, the flatness factor for the right and left eye is 2.00 D. Do not go beyond −2.00 D.

Type of drill: Modified Preliminary Drill

29.1.2 ANISOMETROPIA

29.1.2.1 MODERATE AND MIDRANGE

- For example, OD –1.00 D, OS –2.25 D

There is a disparity of at least −1.00 D, when one eye is in the moderate range (−1.00 D to −1.75 D), and the other eye is in the midrange (−2.00 D to −2.75 D). The flatness factor for the right and left lens is 2.00 D flatter than the curvature of the cornea determined at mid K regardless of the weaker eye's prescription (within the midrange). In the above example, the flatness factor would be OD 2.00 D and OS 2.00 D flatter than the curvature of the cornea determined at mid K.

Type of drill: Modified Preliminary Drill

29.1.2.2 MILD AND MODERATE RANGE

- For example, OD –0.50 D, OS –1.50 D

There is a disparity of at least −1.00 D when one eye is in the mild range (−0.50 D to −0.75 D), and the other eye is in the moderate range (−1.00 D to −1.75 D). The flatness factor for the right and left lens is equal to the absolute value of the weaker eye. In the above example, the flatness factor would be OD 1.50 D and OS 1.50 D flatter than the curvature of the cornea determined at mid K.

Type of drill: Modified Preliminary Drill

29.1.3   ANISOMETROPIA AND ASTIGMATISM

29.1.3.1   MODERATE AND MIDRANGE ANISOMETROPIA AND ASTIGMATISM

- For example, OD −1.00 − 1.50 × 180 and OS 2.25 − 1.00 × 180

There is a disparity of at least −1.00 D (or −0.75 D in some cases) when one eye is in the moderate range (−1.00 D to −1.75 D), and the other eye is in the midrange (−2.00 D to −2.75 D). The cylinder in the right eye is over 100% of the sphere. The flatness factor for the right and left lens is equal to maximum flatness factor. In the above example, the lens' flatness would be OD 2.00 D and OS 2.00 D flatter than the curvature of the cornea determined at mid K. (The maximum flatness factor is 2.00 D.)

Type of drill: Modified Preliminary Drill

29.1.3.2   MILD AND MODERATE ANISOMETROPIA AND ASTIGMATISM

- For example, OD −0.75 − 1.50 × 180 and OS − 1.75 − 0.75 × 180

There is a disparity of at least −1.00 D (or −0.75 D in some cases) when one eye is in the mild range (−0.50 D to −0.75 D) and the other eye is in the moderate range (−1.00 D to −1.75 D). The cylinder in the right eye is over 100% of the sphere. The flatness factor for the right and left lens is equal to the absolute value of the weaker eye. In the above example, the flatness factor would be OD 1.75 D and OS 1.75 D flatter than the curvature of the cornea determined at mid K.

Type of drill: Modified Preliminary Drill.

29.1.4 MILD MYOPIA AND ASTIGMATISM

The flatness factor and thickness for a "plano" lens in relation to mild myopia and astigmatism are as follows.

29.1.4.1 MILD MYOPIA AND ASTIGMATISM −0.25 D TO −1.00 D

- If you have mild myopia (−0.50 D to −0.75 D) and your cylinder is from −0.25 D to −1.00 D, the flatness factor is equal to the absolute value of the sphere. If the sphere is −0.50 D or −0.75 D, the flatness of the plain contact lens should be, respectively, 0.50 D or 0.75 D flatter than the curvature of the cornea determined at mid K. The thickness is 0.15 mm.

Type of drill: Apply the Standard Drill if the cylinder is −0.25 D. Apply the Modified Preliminary Drill for a cylinder 0.50 D and over. Perform a resistance test in borderline cases such as −0.50 − 0.25 × 180 especially if the prescription is for both eyes.

29.1.4.2 MILD MYOPIA AND ASTIGMATISM −1.25 D TO −2.00 D

- If you have mild myopia (−0.50 D to −0.75 D) and your cylinder is −1.25 D to −2.00 D, the flatness factor is equal to the absolute value of the sphere plus 0.25 D. If the sphere is −0.50 D or −0.75 D, the flatness of the plain contact lens should be, respectively, 0.75 D or 1.00 D flatter than the curvature of your cornea determined at mid K. The thickness is 0.15 mm.

Type of drill: Modified Preliminary Drill

29.1.4.3 Mild Myopia AND ASTIGMATISM OVER −2.00 D

- If you have mild myopia (−0.50 D to −0.75 D) and your cylinder is over −2.00 D, the flatness factor is different. It would be dealt with in another publication on treating difficult cases of myopia.

29.3.4   MODERATE MYOPIA AND ASTIGMATISM

The flatness factor and thickness for a "plano" lens in relation to moderate myopia and astigmatism are as follows:

29.3.4.1   MODERATE MYOPIA AND ASTIGMATISM −0.25 D TO −1.00 D

- If you have moderate myopia (−1.00 D to −1.75 D) and your cylinder is from −0.25 D to −1.00 D, the flatness factor is equal to the absolute value of the sphere. If the sphere is −1.00 D, −1.25 D, −1.50 D, or −1.75 D, the flatness of the plain contact lens should be, respectively, 1.00 D, 1.25 D, 1.50 D, or 1.75 D flatter than the curvature of your cornea determined at mid K. The thickness is 0.15 mm.

Type of drill: Apply the Standard Drill for a cylinder up to −0.50 D. Apply the Modified Preliminary Drill for a cylinder 0.75 D and over. Perform a resistance test in borderline cases such as $-1.00 - 0.50 \times 180$.

29.3.4.2   MODERATE MYOPIA AND ASTIGMATISM −1.25 D TO −2.00 D

- If you have moderate myopia (−1.00 D to −1.75 D) and your cylinder is from −1.25 D to −2.00 D, the flatness factor is equal to the absolute value of the sphere plus 0.25 D. If the sphere is −1.00 D, −1.25 D, −1.50 D, or −1.75 D, the flatness of the plain contact lens should be, respectively, 1.25 D, 1.50 D, 1.75 D, or 2.00 D flatter than the curvature of your cornea determined at mid K. The thickness is 0.15 mm.

Type of drill: Modified Preliminary Drill

29.3.4.3   MODERATE MYOPIA AND ASTIGMATISM OVER −2.00

- If you have moderate myopia and your cylinder is over −2.00 D, the flatness factor is different. It would be dealt with in another publication on treating difficult cases of myopia.

Diopters to Millimeters of Radius

Diopters	mm	Diopters	mm	Diopters	mm	Diopters	mm	Diopters	mm
48.15	7.01	44.94	7.51	42.13	8.01	39.66	8.51	37.46	9.01
48.08	7.02	44.88	7.52	42.08	8.02	39.61	8.52	37.42	9.02
48.01	7.03	44.82	7.53	42.03	8.03	39.57	8.53	37.38	9.03
47.94	7.04	44.76	7.54	41.98	8.04	39.52	8.54	37.33	9.04
47.87	7.05	44.70	7.55	41.93	8.05	39.47	8.55	37.29	9.05
47.80	7.06	44.64	7.56	41.87	8.06	39.43	8.56	37.25	9.06
47.74	7.07	44.58	7.57	41.82	8.07	39.38	8.57	37.21	9.07
47.67	7.08	44.53	7.58	41.77	8.08	39.34	8.58	37.17	9.08
47.60	7.09	44.47	7.59	41.72	8.09	39.29	8.59	37.13	9.09
47.54	7.10	44.41	7.60	41.67	8.10	39.24	8.60	37.09	9.10
47.47	7.11	44.35	7.61	41.62	8.11	39.20	8.61	37.05	9.11
47.40	7.12	44.29	7.62	41.56	8.12	39.15	8.62	37.01	9.12
47.34	7.13	44.23	7.63	41.51	8.13	39.11	8.63	36.97	9.13
47.27	7.14	44.18	7.64	41.46	8.14	39.06	8.64	36.93	9.14
47.20	7.15	44.12	7.65	41.41	8.15	39.02	8.65	36.89	9.15
47.14	7.16	44.06	7.66	41.36	8.16	38.97	8.66	36.84	9.16
47.07	7.17	44.00	7.67	41.31	8.17	38.93	8.67	36.80	9.17
47.01	7.18	43.95	7.68	41.26	8.18	38.88	8.68	36.76	9.18
46.94	7.19	43.89	7.69	41.21	8.19	38.84	8.69	36.72	9.19
46.88	7.20	43.83	7.70	41.16	8.20	38.79	8.70	36.68	9.20
46.81	7.21	43.77	7.71	41.11	8.21	38.75	8.71	36.64	9.21
46.75	7.22	43.72	7.72	41.06	8.22	38.70	8.72	36.61	9.22
46.68	7.23	43.66	7.73	41.01	8.23	38.66	8.73	36.57	9.23
46.62	7.24	43.60	7.74	40.96	8.24	38.62	8.74	36.53	9.24
46.55	7.25	43.55	7.75	40.91	8.25	38.57	8.75	36.49	9.25
46.49	7.26	43.49	7.76	40.86	8.26	38.53	8.76	36.45	9.26
46.42	7.27	43.44	7.77	40.81	8.27	38.48	8.77	36.41	9.27
46.36	7.28	43.38	7.78	40.76	8.28	38.44	8.78	36.37	9.28
46.30	7.29	43.32	7.79	40.71	8.29	38.40	8.79	36.33	9.29
46.23	7.30	43.27	7.80	40.66	8.30	38.35	8.80	36.29	9.30
46.17	7.31	43.21	7.81	40.61	8.31	38.31	8.81	36.25	9.31
46.11	7.32	43.16	7.82	40.56	8.32	38.27	8.82	36.21	9.32
46.04	7.33	43.10	7.83	40.52	8.33	38.22	8.83	36.17	9.33
45.98	7.34	43.05	7.84	40.47	8.34	38.18	8.84	36.13	9.34
45.92	7.35	42.99	7.85	40.42	8.35	38.14	8.85	36.10	9.35
45.86	7.36	42.94	7.86	40.37	8.36	38.09	8.86	36.06	9.36
45.79	7.37	42.88	7.87	40.32	8.37	38.05	8.87	36.02	9.37

Diopters	mm	Diopters	mm	Diopters	mm	Diopters	mm	Diopters	mm
45.73	7.38	42.83	7.88	40.27	8.38	38.01	8.88	35.98	9.38
45.67	7.39	42.78	7.89	40.23	8.39	37.96	8.89	35.94	9.39
45.61	7.40	42.72	7.90	40.18	8.40	37.92	8.90	35.90	9.40
45.55	7.41	42.67	7.91	40.13	8.41	37.88	8.91	35.87	9.41
45.49	7.42	42.61	7.92	40.08	8.42	37.84	8.92	35.83	9.42
45.42	7.43	42.56	7.93	40.04	8.43	37.79	8.93	35.79	9.43
45.36	7.44	42.51	7.94	39.99	8.44	37.75	8.94	35.75	9.44
45.30	7.45	42.45	7.95	39.94	8.45	37.71	8.95	35.71	9.45
45.24	7.46	42.40	7.96	39.89	8.46	37.67	8.96	35.68	9.46
45.18	7.47	42.35	7.97	39.85	8.47	37.63	8.97	35.64	9.47
45.12	7.48	42.29	7.98	39.80	8.48	37.58	8.98	35.60	9.48
45.06	7.49	42.24	7.99	39.75	8.49	37.54	8.99	35.56	9.49
45.00	7.50	42.19	8.00	39.71	8.50	37.50	9.00	35.53	9.50

KEYWORDS

- prescription
- diopters
- millimeter of radius
- thickness
- diameter
- material
- flatness factor

ADDENDUM

The following information was mainly written for your patients. You can relay to them any topic you think is relevant. Emphasis is placed on contact lens insertion and removal, how to apply the plunger, and relaxing the eye to address progressive myopia or a partial resistance.

RANGE OF MYOPIA

Mild myopia is from −0.25 D to −0.75 D. Moderate nearsightedness is from −1.00 D to −1.75 D. These classifications were not just based on what the patients in general can or cannot see prior to ortho C. The expected outcome, retention period, and how long it took to achieve the proper retention after ortho C was also taken into account.

CONVERSION FROM SNELLEN CHART READING TO DIOPTER

Your visual acuity is a measure of the finest detail you can see. The measurements are made with a Snellen chart. The specific line of letters which you can see is indicated at the margin. Line 8 is the 20/20 line. If you have 20/20 vision, it means that you can read the 20/20 line on the Snellen chart at 20 ft away. If you have 20/40 vision, it means that you can only read the 20/40 line at 20 ft, whereas a person with normal vision can see it at 40 ft, etc.

Your prescription, on the other hand, is expressed in diopters. A diopter represents the optical power of a lens; the higher the dioptric value, the stronger the prescription. A negative value is assigned to it if you are nearsighted to denote that it is a minus or concave lens. (If you are farsighted, it is a plus lens or convex lens.)

The following is a conversion from the readings on a Snellen chart to approximate measurements expressed in diopters:

Snellen Chart	Line Diopter Correction
20/20	0.00
20/30	−0.50
20/40	−0.75
20/50	−1.00
20/70	−1.25
20/100	−1.50
20/150	−2.00
20/200	−2.50
20/250	−3.00

The above table is for information only. When you read a Snellen chart at 20 ft away, the above conversion to diopters is an approximation without taking into account the ability of the crystalline lens to assist the eye to see better. The actual results also depends on the setting (whether there is natural light present or artificial light or hardly any light), how the measurements are taken (with a phoropter or trial lenses), and whether the patient was "fogged."

THE K READING

The curvature of your cornea must be obtained before you can be fitted with an ortho C lens. It is determined by an instrument call a keratometer. The keratometer readings (or K readings, as it is often called) are expressed in diopters. Two separate readings are required: the horizontal curvature and the vertical curvature. With these measurements, you can then calculate the mid K.

The mid K refers to the average of the horizontal and vertical curvatures. For example, if your horizontal reading is 42.00 D, and your vertical reading is 43.00 D, then your mid K is 42.50 D. Given the above K readings, a lens 1.00 D flatter than the curvature of your cornea at mid K is not as flat as a lens 1.00 D flatter than the bottom K. If a lens was determined at 1.00 D from the bottom K, or the flatter K, which happens to be 42.00 D in this case, it means that it would actually depress the top K, or the steeper K, by 2.0 D. That amount of depression may interfere with the draw of the lens. You would sometimes see a blur spot on your contact lens if it is too flat. It is the area where the higher curvature of your cornea comes into contact with the lens. Thus, it is better to use the mid K to determine the flatness of the contact lens.

The difference between the horizontal and vertical curvature represents one type of astigmatism called corneal astigmatism. Corneal astigmatism is a refractive error due to the irregularity of the cornea, and it is a common characteristic with almost every cornea. A drop of solution onto the lens prior to insertion smooths out the cornea by filling in the ripples caused by the difference in curvature. It allows an even "contact lens draw."

VISUAL ACUITY TEST

Line 8 (the D E F P O T E C line) is the standard 20/20 line on all Snellen charts. The chart in this book is calibrated for 10 ft. Mark that spot on the floor. It indicates where you would stand for a visual acuity test. Hang the chart by an incoming source of natural light. If you are not close to a window that allows natural lighting, then hang the chart in adequate artificial lighting. The room should be well lit so that minor changes in visual acuity would be noticeable.

In a setting illuminated by natural light the 20/20 line or line 8 represents your normal vision during the day when you are outdoors. If line 9 (the 20/15 line) or line 10 (the 20/13 line) comes into focus, it represents normal vision in dim lighting, artificial lighting, and outdoors at night. The aperture opens more under those conditions.

You may need a pair of weaker glasses if you have a partial resistance. If it is required for the blackboard or driving during the day, then it is sufficient for the glasses to correct the visual acuity to 20/25 (line 7) or even 20/30 (line 6). If it is also required for driving at night, then you need another pair to correct the visual acuity to 20/15 or 20/13 (line 9 or line 10) depending on the requirements. You just need the following pairs of glasses in your inventory: −0.25 D, −0.50 D, −0.75 D, and −1.00 D.

Check the binocular and monocular visual acuity. When you are checking each eye, cover the other eye, but keep the covered eye open. For some individuals, especially with anisometropic amblyopia, it takes a lot of effort to close one eye and read with the other. When occluding the eye, leave a gap by holding the palm 2–3 in. away to prevent instrument myopia. It is normal for each eye with primary refractive error to see one line less compared to what you can see with both eyes. (Refer to the chapter *The Procedure* for an explanation.)

Record what line you can see with both eyes and with each eye: line 3, line 4, etc. If it is line 4 plus two letters on the next line, then record that as line 4 + 2, etc. If it is line 4 plus three letters on line 5, then record that as line 5 − 2. It is written as 5 − 2 instead of 4 + 3. Line 5 is more predominant since you can read more than half the letters on that line. If you read less than half the letters on that line, then less emphasis would be given to line 5.

In Canada, the requirement for driving with a general license without glasses is a visual acuity of 20/50 (line 4). In most of the states in the United States, it is a visual acuity of 20/40 (line 5) in the better eye. But at night, the aperture opens more; and similar to the wider opening of the lens on a camera, an image in the distance becomes blurred. Thus, one pair of glasses should be fitted for the day and another pair for the nighttime. Otherwise the nighttime glasses would be overcorrected in the day.

PROVIDE A VISUAL AID IN THE INTERIM

In the short term, provide a reduced prescription such as −0.25 D, −0.50 D, or −0.75 D for clients with mild or moderate myopia with a partial resistance. The visual aid would only be worn to help make out objects in the distance in low or dim lighting situations. In the daytime, the client's visual acuity is okay. Offsetting strain is exemplified in how glasses should be prescribed for severe myopia to prevent progressive myopia. One pair should be given during the day and another pair at night for driving (and another pair for working in front of a computer screen if necessary). After treating my severe myopia (of −10.00 D), for example, I wear a −1.25 D pair of glasses during the day and a −2.00 D pair of glasses at night when I drive. I do not need any visual aid for the midrange (in front of a computer screen).

A weaker prescription may be required in the short term due to the following:

- The aperture of the eye opens wider at night due to the lack of light. Thus objects in the distance are a bit blurred if the eye still has a partial resistance.

- The eyeball offers more resistance than the crystalline lens. It may take a bit longer to reverse the myopic shape of the eyeball if it deviated more than usual compared to the lens.

- The eye may not totally conform to the myopic model. It puts up a higher resistance if the patient was subjected to certain extraneous variables.

NEED A FEW DROPS PRIOR TO INSERTION

It is critical to place a drop of contact lens solution onto the lens before insertion. The solution transmits the influence from the ortho C lens to your eye. The extra layer of liquid serves as an artificial cornea. It fills the unevenness on the cornea due to cornea astigmatism and allows the "contact lens draw" to be even along the perimeter of the lens. Otherwise the treatment may not work properly; and in some cases, it may not work at all.

Some eye care specialists would tell their patients to place a minimal amount of solution on the rigid lens, or rub the solution onto the lens, or even take the lens out of the container without adding any solution since it is already soaked with solution. Those instructions were intended for normal wear with a conventional lens, not for ortho C. Instead, place a drop of conditioning solution onto the cavity of the lens until it fills up to the brim. It should form a hump once it fills up the well of the lens. Now it is ready for insertion.

INSERTION

Balance the lens on top of your index finger. Position it as close to the tip of your finger as possible. At first, you may spill a fair amount of the solution just trying to balance it on your finger (or the lens will slip off before it makes contact with the cornea); but with practice, as you perform the movement more smoothly, you will retain most or all of the solution.

If you are right handed, balance the lens on the right index finger. Then separate the upper and lower lids. Place your left middle finger on the upper lid and pull up and anchor it against the upper eye socket. Then place your right middle finger on the lower lid and pull down at the same time and anchor it against the lower eye socket. Then insert the lens that you balanced on top of your right index finger by lightly touching the hump of contact lens solution onto your cornea.

You are actually making contact with the contact lens solution first. It is the meniscus that pulls the lens onto your eye. You do not have to jam the lens in. Keep that in mind, and it would reduce the fear of lens insertion.

Continue to practice overcoming the urge to close your eye at the last minute. Do not get into the habit of throwing the lens into your eye as quick as you can and hope that you can beat your blink. A better alternative is to lean the lens onto the cornea by making contact with the bottom half first. The meniscus assists by pulling in the upper half of the lens. The insertion is one smooth movement to minimize or prevent spillage. Then you release the lower lid first and then the upper lid. Repeat the same procedure with the other eye. You would use the same hand to insert the lens.

REMOVING THE LENS

WHY A PLUNGER

Most people can remove a hard prescription contact lens by conventional means—by pulling the ends of the upper and lower eyelids with your index and middle finger to pop it out—which your eye care specialist would gladly demonstrate for you. It is the normal way to remove a hard lens; but because the lens I am recommending is flexible, it is a more difficult procedure. There is the tendency to exert more force to remove an ortho C lens compared to a conventional lens because the lens hugs closer to the cornea. The area near the flange of a flexible lens adheres to your cornea more readily. There is less gap between the contact lens and the cornea for the lids to wedge between them.

A contact lens plunger (or contact lens remover) can save you a lot of aggravation. You can purchase it from some optical outlets or you can even order it online. It is about an inch and a half in length. The whole unit, the suction cup and the shaft, is made of rubber. It is designed to remove a rigid contact lens. It also works on a flexible ortho C lens, but do not use it on a soft contact lens. It will adhere onto the cornea as well as the lens since a soft contact lens is very thin and the material is very pliable.

STANDARD PLUNGER

It is important to see the lens before you attempt to remove it. The lens may shift at the last minute. Look for the outline or the rim of the contact lens. It becomes more visible if you stand in front of a washroom mirror and let the lights from the fixture reflect off the edge of the lens. Turn your head side to side and up and down until it comes into view.

Line up the suction cup over the center of the contact lens and touch it lightly. Then gently pull the plunger half an inch away from the cornea. If the suction cup does not stick onto the lens, wet it with contact lens solution and try again. Remember to pull gently to cover a distance half an inch to an inch from the cornea in case the lens shifted at the last minute. (Refer to the section In Case You Miss below.)

HOLLOW PLUNGER

Another type of plunger is a hollow plunger. It has a hole extending from the middle of the cup up along the shaft. You have to squeeze the handle slightly while you apply the cup onto the lens. Allow the cup to sit on the lens for a few seconds before you release the grip. This creates the suction. To release the lens squeeze on the handle again to relieve the suction. Wet the cup before applying it onto the lens if necessary. Once you become proficient in removing the lens with this type of plunger, you would able to touch the lens, release the pressure, create the suction, and pull all in one motion to remove the lens.

IN CASE YOU MISS

There may be the rare occasion when the suction cup comes into contact with the "white of the eye" when you miss the lens, or it may come into contact with the cornea when the lens shifted at the last minute and you are not aware of it. It rarely happens, but when it does the cup will adhere securely onto the eye.

Do not yank on the plunger. The excessive force may rip the first layer of the cornea if the lens shifted and the plunger came into contact with the cornea. There are five layers. The first layer can regenerate after a day, but there would be pain due to photophobia. It is painful to expose the eye to light. You have to keep it covered.

With a solid plunger, slide the plunger toward the corner of your eye and rotate it off. It will easily come off. The curvature of the sclera near the cornea is different and that allows air to seep in to relieve the suction.

With a plunger with a hole in the middle, all you have to do is squeeze the handle again. This will release the suction. Thus, this type of plunger is more safe than the other type. In some cases, you may still have to slide the plunger toward the corner of the eye where the curvature is different. It allows more air into the cup and the plunger should come off.

REMOVAL WITH CHEWING GUM

A plunger will eventually start to lose its suction, so keep a spare one. If both of them were misplaced and you did not realize it when you wore the lens, chewing gum can be used as a last resort (apart from the conventional method of removal). I know. It sounds pretty gruesome since saliva has bacteria, but we are talking about first aid. There is a tradeoff between alleviating the discomfort of having a lens on your eye and the remote chance of eye infection. So here is what you do:

Chew the gum until most of the flavor is gone. By then, it should stick readily onto the lens. Roll the gum up into an oblong shape. Tap one end onto the lens and wait for about 10 s for the gum to displace the tears and adhere onto the lens. Then give it a slight pull.

You may have to make several attempts before it sticks onto the lens. The contact lens material is porous, and the surface will be saturated with tears. If you have trouble adhering the gum onto the lens, here is what you do: stop blinking. Each time you blink, you generate tears. Dry the surface of the lens by dabbing it with the tip of a rolled up kleenex. Then try again—without blinking.

CONVENTIONAL REMOVAL

If you misplaced the plunger (and there is no gum), a conventional way of removal is in order. It may take a bit longer to wedge the lids between the lens and the cornea. The design of the lens allows it to hug the cornea closer than a conventional rigid gas permeable lens (RGP) lens, but the lens should eventually come out if you apply the following method (after the solution drains and the meniscus pulls less on the lens to increase the gap between the flange of the lens and the corner.

In most cases, the upper lid is attached to the upper third of the lens. Most lenses I designed are upper lid attachment. Open the eye wide and position the upper lid over the top of the lens with the index finger from one hand. At the same time position the lower lid against the bottom part of the lens with the index finger from the other hand. Then pull the upper and lower lid outwards toward the corner of the eye to wedge it into the gap. The lens should pop out.

EMERGENCY REMOVAL

The lens can sometime become "sucked on" if you accidentally push against it by rubbing your eye. It is like two wet plates stuck together when one is on top of the other. The lens can also adhere onto your cornea if you fell asleep with the lens on or if you apply the wrong type of contact lens solution (solution intended for soft lens instead of a rigid lens).

Do not go to the Emergency Ward right away. From the reports some of my patients gave, their methods involved different ways to pry the lens out. It will rip the first layer of the cornea in the process. To remove the lens, perform the following instead:

Pull down on the lower lid slightly with the index finger. Apply several drops of rigid contact lens solution to the well of the lid. Then blink for a few times. Wait for about 30 s for the solution will soak through the porous lens. Then try to remove it gently with the plunger. Depending on how long the lens was "sucked on," most likely it would not come out after the first attempt. You may have to repeat the above steps three or four times before the lens would come off.

CLEANING THE LENS

Rinse the lenses in warm tap water to clean the tears and loose protein before you place it back into the soaking solution. Use warm water. Not hot. The lens is thin, and it can easily become warped if you run hot water over it. Leave the lenses immersed in the soaking solution since it contains disinfectant which will deal with any impurities in the water. It also keeps them hydrated to prevent dry spots. Do not store the ortho C lenses dry if

300   Addendum

you intend to use them regularly. Dry spots can interfere with the "contact lens draw."

Make sure you have the correct contact solution for RGP lens. It should be written on the label that it is for RGP lenses. Do not use soft contact lens solution for insertion. The lens will adhere to the cornea.

A multiaction solution will have cleaning agents to remove the protein. A bottle of soaking solution that does not have a protein remover should have another bottle of cleaning solution included in the package. The cleaning liquid is white to distinguish it from the soaking solution.

Clean the lenses regularly with the cleaning solution once every couple of months or so. Apply a drop on the top and bottom of the lens and gently rub it on the palm in a swirling motion for 10 s or so. Then rinse the lens in warm water. Then deposit the lenses in the new soaking solution.

You should change the soaking solution in the container more frequently to decrease the risk of eye infection. The solution is stagnant, and it is an ideal culture for breeding bacteria. Change it about every 2 weeks regardless of your wearing schedule to avoid contamination.

Clean the contact lens case thoroughly. It is a good idea to replace it after six months with a new one. The other option is to immerse it in boiling water for half a minute and then clean it thoroughly afterwards.

TYPES OF SOLUTION

There are two types of contact lens solution made by Boston for rigid contact lens: Boston Advance and Boston Simplus. You will find the solution thicker than soft contact lens solution. Never use soft contact lens solution on a rigid lens. The solution would drain immediately and the lens would end up adhering to the eye. (Refer to the section on Emergency Removal.)

PALMING

PURPOSE

The drill is intended to relax the ciliary muscle. It also reminds the upper lid not to bear heavily down against the cornea by squinting whenever there is something blur. It attempts to change the habit of trying to see everything sharp. It reminds you to "let go" of a blur object in the distance and accept it as it is.

HOW TO PALM

Perform the drill without any lenses on. Start by resting your elbows on the table. Keep your back straight. The table should not be so low that it forces you to hunch over. Maintaining a proper posture helps your body to relax, and that in turn assists in stimulating the ciliary muscle to relax. When you close your eyes, you do not have to squeeze the lids tightly to keep them shut. When you cover them with the palms of your hands, your palms act as a second pair of lids to induce a higher sense of relaxation by reducing the effort it takes to keep your lids closed.

Cup your hands and rest the heel of each palm on your cheekbone. The palms of your hands do not come into contact with the lids of your eyes. Form an inverted "V" with the edge of both of your hands by overlapping the fingers of one hand over the top of the fingers of your other hand, and wedge the middle of the "V" on top of the bridge of your nose. The thumbs rest along the corner and the top of your eye sockets along the eye brows to assist in anchoring the hands. Relax your fingers to further stimulate the muscles of your eyes to relax. But do not be so relax that your fingers become mushy. You still want to maintain the cupped position of your hands. Experiment to find which hand should overlap the other without producing too much discomfort.

Your mind should be blank. Do not think about anything. There should be total darkness. After a while, some thoughts may creep in. Do not resist them. Let them appear. Consider them briefly, and then dismiss them. Turn off the lights again, so to speak, and contemplate on total darkness. Later, other thoughts will appear. Again, consider them briefly and dismiss them. Think of the darkness instead. Gradually, its duration will become longer and longer. The intensity of the darkness is synonymous with your ability to relax.

WHEN TO PALM

It should be performed for 2 min or longer before you engage in anything strenuous such as working in front of a computer monitor all day. Palm your eyes after extensive work looking into the distance such as copying notes from the blackboard. When you feel that fatigue is about to set in, take a break and palm your eyes. Do not palm your eyes before or after you perform any ortho C drill. The message sent to the ciliary muscle can interfere with the correct neurological message from the drill, but palming can be done at any other time.

HOW IT BENEFITS YOU

Palming relaxes your eyes by removing the "effort to see" completely (since you are not focusing on anything in particular). It reminds you that there is an on/off switch and you control it. If you leave it in the "on" position all the time, it contributes to "strain." It may cause other ailments as well. It is comparable to always leaving your living room lights on. Sooner or later all of them will burn out.

SWINGING DRILL

PURPOSE

The drill is also intended to relax the ciliary muscle. It reminds you to "let go" of a blur object. It attempts to restore the eye's saccadic movement.

HOW TO PERFORM THE DRILL

Hold a pencil in front of you at arm's length. Swing your head back and forth to the right and then to the left and then to the right, etc. Do it about 30 times at a rate of 1 s per swing. When you swing to the right, the pencil seems to swing to the left, and when you swing to the left, the pencil seems to swing to the right, etc. Do not look at the pencil. Swing right past it. When you swing your head to one side, it is 30° away. Do not swing 180°. Swing in a relaxed motion. There is no effort involved at all.

STRETCHING DRILLS

ADJUSTING THE READING RANGE

Reduce near-point stress by adjusting the reading range to 14 or 16 in. away. If you have severe myopia you may not be able to maintain that range immediately. To break the habit of reading too close, you have to gradually replace it with another habit. Consciously "stretch" your vision within that distance and hold it for half a minute or so. Do not try to maintain the stretch too long or too often to avoid triggering an excessive "effort to see."

ADJUSTING THE COMPUTER RANGE

The same idea applies to working in front of a computer. The ideal working distance is about 20 in. away from the monitor. To make the drill more practical, maintain a distance 16–20 in. away. Consciously "stretch" your vision within that distance and hold it for half a minute or so. Do not try to maintain the stretch too long or too often to avoid triggering an excessive "effort to see."

Perform the "stretching" drill two or three times a day. After the drill, let the vision settle to its natural range which is a bit closer. Gradually, you will be able to adopt the preferred range longer. (Refer to the chapter *The Effort to See* for more information.)

LET GO BY WATCHING TV

The more nearsighted you are, the more your saccadic range would recede. The scanning area shrinks as the saccadic movement becomes more sluggish. It affects your ability to "let go" of a blur object.

The TV is a very effective tool to train you to "let go" and accept a blur image by activating the saccadic movement. It improves the ability to look away instead of constantly straining to bring an object into focus. You do not have to worry about what to do after you "let go" of an image that is too blur. You will be preoccupied with the next frame which will automatically present another image that allows your vision to rest (when it easily comes into focus), or another image that is also too blur (and you also have to "let go" of it).

Sit at a comfortable distance from the TV without any visual aid. When an image comes into focus by means of a "focal point draw," it will disappear from the TV screen just as quickly since the picture keeps changing. There is no guarantee that the next image will also produce a "focal point draw." Even if you do not "let go" in time, the rate which each image changes on the TV screen will assist in disengaging from central focus mode. Thus it trains you to "let go" subconsciously. But if you keep making a conscious effort to "let go" when you do not "let go" in time (when a movie is "slow going"), sit closer to the TV to avoid fatigue.

Once you learn to "let go" of a blur image subconsciously, you are actually taking a rest in between "focal point draws," and that is what makes an "intermittent draw" less demanding compared to a "continuous draw." A "draw" becomes continuous if you do not let go of a blur object. It is continuous even if that object does not come into focus. You will keep trying to consciously force it into focus. After you perform the TV drill for a few weeks, the "draw" will become intermittent. The goal is to become less and less conscious of the whole process.

When you perform the ortho C drills regularly, it will relax the ciliary muscles sufficiently to allow you to keeping up with the rate the picture changes on the screen. When the myopic eye's saccadic movement is brought up to speed, you will automatically relax and either allow a "focal point draw" to take place or ignore the object that is in question. You do not have to think about which choice to make. I am not saying that you should never be conscious of bringing a distant image into focus. You can do it once in a while, but it becomes tiring if you do it all the time.

As your vision improves, you can move a bit farther from the TV. You can also perform the "stretching" drill with the TV. Do not try to maintain the stretch too long to avoid triggering an excessive "effort to see." After about 5 min, go back to the normal range. (Refer to the chapter *The Effort to See* for more information.)

DO NOT COMBINE THE RELAXATION EXERCISES WITH ANY ORTHO C DRILLS

The palming, swinging, and stretching drills can be performed regularly, but do not perform them prior or after any ortho C drills. The natural relaxation exercises will become an extraneous variable because they neurologically interfere with the neurological message reinstated by an ortho C drill.

THE 20/20 RULE

You do not have to avoid near or close up work to maintain your improved visual acuity. If you adhere to the 20/20 rule, you should do just fine because the eye is made to work. The 20/20 rule states that after 20 min, take a break by looking away beyond 20 ft for 20 s.

At first you can set a timer. Later it becomes a habit. You may not look away exactly at 20-min intervals, but you would still look away to relax—even if it is 5 ft away.

HYPOTHESES

ON THE PROBLEM

The motor cortex regards the myopic eye to be in near focus mode due to the excessive tightness of the oblique muscles. It maintains the myopic shape of the crystalline lens and eyeball even when the eye attempts to make out an object far away.

ON THE TREATMENT

When a "contact lens draw" is combined with a "focal point draw," it triggers a reversal in myopia by "loosening" the oblique muscles. When the shapes of the lens and eyeball are not restricted by the tension of the oblique muscles, the brain considers the eye to be emmetropic. It stimulates the eye neurologically to correct itself. The process is the reverse of near-point stress.

THEORIES

ON THE PROBLEM

The first theory on the relationship between the oblique muscles and ciliary muscle of the myopic eye can be expressed as follows: the excessive tension of the oblique muscles causes the ciliary muscle to become tense to entice the crystalline lens to bulge. (The first part of the Preliminary

Drill presupposes that such a condition exists. The drill would not work if the condition did not exist.)

The second theory on the relationship between the oblique muscles and the rectus muscles of the myopic eye can be stated as follows: the excessive tension of the oblique muscle causes the rectus muscles to relax to entice the eyeball to elongate. (The second part of the Standard Drill presupposes that such a condition exists. The drill would not work if the condition did not exist.)

The third theory on the synchronization of the two dual relationships of the myopic eye can be expressed as follows: the tendency for the crystalline lens to bulge also causes the eye to elongate. The third part of the Standard Drill presupposes that such a condition exists. The drill would not work if the condition did not exist.

ON THE TREATMENT

Prior to ortho C, the motor cortex ignores the myopee's perception of a distant object even though the subject knows that it is far away. Due to the tension of the oblique muscles, the brain interprets the eye to be in near focus mode. It bypasses the neurosensory message of a blur distant object. When a "contact lens draw" combines with a "focal point draw," it expands the vertical height and horizontal width of the eye (when viewing the eye from the front). It "loosens" the oblique muscles' grip around the eyeball. The visual cortex will then take the subject's depth perception of a distant image into account. It recognizes that the eye is in distant focus mode. The motor cortex reinstates the correct neuromuscular message to allow distant objects to come into focus. (Refer to the chapter *How It Reverses Nearsightedness*.)

REFERENCES

Barnes, J. *Improve Your Eye Sight*; Souvenir Press Ltd.: London, UK, 1999.

Bailey, M. D.; Sinnott, L. T.; Mutti, D. O. Ciliary Body Thickness and Refractive Error in Children. *Invest. Ophthalmol. Vis. Sci.* **2008,** *49* (10), 4353–4360.

Caban, D. *Hermann von Helmholtz and the Foundations of Nineteenth Century Science*; University of California Press: Berkeley, LA, 1993.

Chornell, G.; Hanebaum, U.; Hauck, K.; Jeffries, D.; Lorimer, B.; MacIvor, I. *Advance Practice 2: Sight Testing*; The Northern Alberta Institute of Technology: Edmonton, AB, 2010.

Dirani, M.; Shekar, S. N.; Baird, P. N. The Role of Education Attainment in Refraction: The Genes in Myopia (GEM) Twin Study. *Invest. Ophthalmol. Vis. Sci.* **2008,** *49* (2), 534–538.

Doonan, B. Model of Visual Focusing Involving Extraocular Muscles and the Causes of Myopia and Glaucoma. *Med. Hypotheses* **1984,** *13* (1), 115–118.

Ghosh, A.; Collins, M. J.; Read, S. A.; Davis, B. A.; Chatterjee, P. Axial Elongation Associated with Biomechanical Factors During Near Work. *Optom. Vis. Sci.* **2014,** *91* (3), 322–329.

Grierson, I. *The Eye Book*; Liverpool University Press: Liverpool, UK, 2000.

Grosvenor, T. Reduction in Axial Length with Age: An Emmetropizing Mechanism for the Adult Eye? *Am. J. Optom. Physiol. Opt.* **1987,** *64* (9), 657–663.

Grosvenor, T. *Primary Care Optometry*; Butterworth-Heinemann: St. Louis, MO, 2007.

Iribarren, R.; Morgan, I. G.; Nangia, V.; Jonas, J. B. Crystalline Lens Power and Refractive Error. *Invest. Ophthalmol. Vis. Sci.* **2012,** *53*, 543–550.

Kuchem, M. K.; Sinnott, L. T.; Kao, C. Y.; Bailey, M. D. Ciliary Muscle Thickness in Anisometropia. *Optom. Vis. Sci.* **2013,** *90* (11), 1312–1320.

Lally, P.; Van Jaarsveld, C. H. M.; Potts, H. W. W.; Wardle, J. How Are Habits Formed: Modelling Habit Formation in the Real World. *Eur. J. Social Psychol.* **2010,** *40* (6), 998–1009.

Liberman, J. *Take Off Your Glasses and See*; Three Rivers Press: New York, NY, 1995.

Muftuoglu, O.; Hosal, B. M.; Zilelioglu, G. Ciliary Body Thickness in Unilateral High Axial Myopia. *Eye* **2009,** *23*, 1176–1181.

Mutti, D. O.; Mitchell, G. L.; Sinnott, L. T.; Jones-Jordan, L. A.; Moeschberger, M. L.; Cotter, S. A.; Kleinstein, R. N.; Manny, R. E.; Twelker, J. D.; Zadnik, K. Corneal and Crystalline Lens Dimensions Before and After Myopia Onset. *Optom. Vis. Sci.* **2012,** *89* (3), 251–262.

Oliveira, C.; Tello, C.; Liebmann, J. M.; Ritch, R. Ciliary Body Thickness Increases with Increasing Axial Myopia. *Am. J. Ophthalmol.* **2005,** *140* (2), 324–325.

Stein, H. A.; Slatt, B. J.; Stein, R. M.; Freeman, M. I. *Fitting Guide for Rigid and Soft Contact Lenses*; Mosby Incorporated: St. Louis, MO, 2002.

Yee, J. W. Correct Mild Myopia by Means of Orthoculogy. *Med. Hypothesis* **2011,** *76* (3), 332–335.

Yee, J. W. Correcting Corneal Astigmatism by Reinstating the Correct Neuromuscular Message. *Med. Hypothesis* **2012,** *79* (3), 368–371.

Yee, J. W. Correcting Lenticular Astigmatism by Reinstating the Correct Neuromuscular Message. *Med. Hypothesis* **2013a,** *81* (1), 36–40.

Yee, J. W. Preventing Retinal Detachment by Averting Asthenopia that Contributes to Progressive Myopia. *OA Med. Hypothesis* **2013b,** *1* (2), 15.

Yee, J. W. Neurological Implications in the Treatment of Myopia by Means of Orthoculogy. *J. Neurol. Neurophysiol.* **2014,** *5*, 257. DOI:10.4172/2155-9562.1000257.

Zadnik, K.; Mutti, D.; Fusaro, R.; Adams, A. Longitudinal Evidence of Crystalline Lens Thinning in Children. *Invest. Ophthalmol. Vis. Sci.* **1995,** *36* (8), 1581–1587.

INTERNATIONAL REVIEWS

I first began wearing glasses to correct nearsightedness when I was 13. Over a period of 44 years and progressively stronger prescriptions, my eyesight declined. Then one day I had a revolutionary idea. What if myopia could be reversed? After much research, I came across a website that explained eye exercises which could correct nearsightedness. I performed these exercises for about a year and my prescription decreased from −4.50 to −2.50. I continued the exercises for another year but could never improve my vision further. That's when I discovered John Yee's concept of orthoculogy.

After only a few months, thanks to Mr. Yee and his lenses, my vision was 20/20. Most optometrists in the United States would believe my results to be impossible. Their unwillingness to consider alternative therapies is surprising, if not downright damaging to patients.

The American Optometric Association (AOA) code of ethics states that a practitioner is obliged to put a patient's welfare above his personal gain and to continually broaden his knowledge of any therapies which might benefit his patient's vision. My own experience with eye care practitioners convinces me that this is frequently not the case.

At the time I began Mr. Yee's therapy, I was told by a local optometrist that anyone who said that I could improve my vision at my age (57) was lying. Fortunately, I didn't listen to that advice. As it turns out, my eyesight got better in spite of optometrists, not because of them.

Recently, I went to get my driver's license renewed and asked to take the vision test to see if I could get the restriction removed. I was quite pleased that I passed. I could see all the way down to the 20/20 line. Mr. Yee's method helped me pass the vision exam.

I'm very grateful that Mr. Yee didn't become discouraged by the lack of acceptance for his ideas. That's usually the way with revolutionary concepts. It takes awhile for them to catch on. I have every confidence that orthoculogy will catch on, and when it does, the eye care profession will be the better for it.

—*N. S. Wikarski, PhD, Florida, United States, Author of The Granite Key,*
Shrouded in Thought, and The Fall of White City

I got to know John over the years as a writer, and we share our general interest as a writer. Later I got to know him as an inventor. I am impressed with his persistent research. He is driven to achieve perfection.

—*Valerie Gyenge, Budapest, Hungary, Olympic gold medalist, 400 m*
freestyle; world record holder, 800 m freestyle, Author of: The Promise, and
The Way They Were, Recipient of the Order of Hungary.

When I started, I could only see line 1 with a pair of −2.00 weaker glasses. Now 6 months later, I can see line 8 with those glasses. The time he spent with me...replacing lenses I broke...shipping problems...somehow we got through it. And we are not finish yet.

—*Sebastian Castenetto, Italy*

I made a special trip to see John at his clinic. He continues to treat me at no cost even after my follow-up visits expired. Eventually, I had the restrictions on my driver's license removed by the Ministry after I past their vision test.

—*Elsa Campuzano, Mexico City, Mexico*

When I first put them on, I was rather amazed that I could see so well because these were plain and not prescription lenses. The optometrist explained that what was probably happening was that my astigmatism was being "masked." Apparently, fluid in the eye fills the gap between the eye and the lens and so improves one's ability to see. But there has to be more to it than that. When I took the lenses off after a few minutes, my vision had changed and I could see better. I was staggered at the result and drove home for the first time in more than a decade without any glasses or lenses.

My vision was so poor beforehand that I struggled to see line 2 on the eye chart. Now I can see line 7, and I am able to drive during the day without lenses of any kind. This is a huge improvement in my vision.

—*Ciaran Ryan, Journalist, Mail and Guardian South Africa,*
Sunday Times, Johannesburg, South Africa

Ortho C follows all the principles of natural vision therapy that I teach my students in qigong. Just like laser surgery, ortho C promises permanent reversal of myopia but with none of the inherent surgical risks of damage to the eye and resulting eyesight. Best of all, it's inexpensive, costing the same as a regular set of prescription glasses—but you don't have to wear them everyday for life! Not only does the price of ortho C makes the treatment available to everyone, but John takes a personal interest in his patients and their improvement in eyesight. Truly a "promising sight for sore eyes"! Thank you John, I can equate your contribution to eye health as what Banting did for diabetes: the affordability of ortho C makes it available to anyone interested in reversing their myopia.

—*Hilda Williams, Edmonton, Alberta, Canada, Professor, Simon Fraser*

I can't thank John Yee enough for what he has done for me. Everything, from our first correspondence until now, his service and care has been way beyond anything I've experienced before. The best of all, though, is that his technique really works better than I could have wished. Before applying the lenses, I was able to read up to and including line 5 on the chart. Now I am able to comfortably read line 7. Prior to this I would not leave the house without my contacts in or my glasses on, I now wear neither. It is such a pleasure not having to bother with contact lenses any more. During the whole time he regularly e-mail me and keep me informed and answer my questions. I wish him all the success in the world for all the help he has provided.

—*Al Stander, Troyeville, Gauteng, South Africa*

Before I started ortho C, my eyesight was around −2.50 D with astigmatism of about −0.50 D. I could not see at all without my glasses. After been in the treatment for a while, I can see a lot better than when I started. I can see almost clearly with a pair of −0.50 D glasses or −0.50 D soft contact lenses. At times, I can see perfectly clear without wearing glasses or contacts.

Something else worth mentioning is John's assistance. Before I went back to Hong Kong, I encountered some problems. John took care of them while I was in Hong Kong. I greatly appreciate his caring service. I feel very happy that I found out about this treatment and I am very much loving the glasses-free world.

—*Florence Leung, RTA, Kowloon, Hong Kong*

At first I was a bit unsure what a method like this could do for me. But my desire to have perfect vision without glasses persisted. I had been wearing glasses pretty much the entire second half of my life. I struggled with my bad habit of forgetting where I left them when I shower sometimes or my bad luck of being hit with the ball in sports with them on. I decided this was worth a try.

To my most pleasant surprise, the ortho C method turned out to be the answer to my prayers! Not only was I able to pass the Ministry of Transportation vision test, but I find that my vision has reached a whole new level. In just after one or two treatment I noticed the improvement in my depth perception. I find that during sunny days there are often many distant objects that seem clear to me. Now, it is beyond 20/20. Furthermore, it has the added benefit of enhancing my hand–eye coordination which has been a real plus in my sports lifestyle. Thank you John, it really was worth "taking a chance" on.

—Kevin Yan, Toronto, Ontario, Canada

John is sincerely interested in my improvement and not just monetary gain. I have not had the pleasure of meeting John face to face but he is trustworthy and has kept in contact via e-mail. I have been receiving treatment from him for a number of years now and I am confident that with his support I can one day achieve the goal of 20/20 vision. This is a very difficult goal to achieve with other opticians/optometrists who are only interested in selling glasses rather than remedying the problem. His charges as a therapist are low. For example: ortho K can charge from $2500 to $3000 for their procedure or laser therapy can go as high as $5000.

I think John is sincere in his therapy, and I wish him luck in it and I hope that he can help me attain my goal of 20/20 vision. I know he will not let me down.

—Zishan Syed, Kent, United Kingdom

You are indeed a very humble person as taught by our Lord. You boast not about your invention, and you do not charge a patient an arm and a leg to provide treatment. I salute you honestly.

—Joseph Yu, BA, MA, ASLA, CLD, OALA, APLD,
Toronto, Ontario, Canada

John assisted my wife and me by e-mail despite we are at the opposite end of the world. We would like to express our deepest gratitude. My wife and I were always hoping that there is a method to deal with myopia effectively. We checked almost all of them out and can say for sure that nothing can compare to the speed of ortho C especially if you have moderate nearsightedness like me. I quickly gained close to 20/20, but he worked with my wife for over a year because she had severe myopia and high astigmatism.

She checked her vision recently, and the results are amazing. Her high astigmatism was reduced, and her vision in each eye has improved by 2 diopters. She now sees line 7 and some of line 8 with a −1.50 pair of glasses. Even her cataracts in both eyes were gone (We don't know for sure if it is because of ortho C or not, but we are inclined to think so.)

—Denis and Liuda Makarov, Penza, Russia

I've been using Dr. Yee's ortho C method to eliminate my reliance on glasses. I started out with a prescription of −1.75 D and high astigmatism of −1.25 D in both eyes. After completing just the first part of the drills, I had to leave (my job requires me to travel a lot). I was still able to see well without glasses in most situations. I just use a pair of −0.50 D glasses when driving and in low light. The progress I've made has been retained over several months and I expect to improve further by the following the rest of the drills. I would recommend this program for anyone with moderate myopia as an alternative to laser surgery.

—Doug McGowan, Edmonds, Washington, United States

Over the course of several months, I have been working with John Yee to improve my severe myopia, I am extremely impressed by the personalized customer service he has offered, even on a daily basis where needed. He has responded to my questions thoughtfully and promptly. He has followed up, in great depth, the basic instructions about his inventive system, offering me a wealth of useful information. This has made the process faster, easier, and more efficacious, allowing me to improve my vision in a remarkably short time frame.

In addition, it has been a pleasure dealing with him, and I am happy to know that I can count on him to assist me in the future for as long as it takes to achieve the degree of improvement I desire. And finally, Mr. Yee has shown remarkable compassion by offering me visual aids at reasonable cost after my health insurance was cancelled due to a job change.

As one of those in the United States who has long admired Canadians' ethics and sense of humanity, I have been pleased to learn how much Mr. Yee embodies those qualities.

—*Sarah M. Eck, Bellevue, Washington, United States*

I am very pleased to hear of John Yee's ethical approach to the dissemination of the specific details of his discovery. He shows the same generosity in his work with students and other individuals who would have difficulty paying for his services. John simply does not charge them. I put a lot of stock in the principle that persons who are fortunate to have knowledge, or special skills, or resources, and reasonable health, should return some of their talent and/or resources to the community. I try to follow this principle, but John Yee exceeds whatever I have been able to do, partly because his approach is so direct and concrete.

—*Dr. Rowland C. Marshall, BA, MA, PhD,*
Chairman, Philosophy Department,
Saint Mary's University, Halifax, Nova Scotia, Canada

ABOUT THE AUTHOR

Pain can drive me to run faster.

—Nikki Kimball, long-distance runner.

John William Yee was born in Glace Bay, Cape Breton, Nova Scotia, Canada. At present, he is conducting research for his doctorate at the University of Liverpool, UK. He received his post master's in Developmental Psychology from Athabasca University, Alberta, Canada. He also graduated from Saint Mary's University, University of Waterloo, Ryerson University, Yorkville University, Northern Alberta Institute of Technology, and Centennial College. He studied psychology, philosophy, economics, mechanical engineering, auto mechanics, and optometry. He is a professor in the optical science faculty at Seneca College.

He has written numerous journal papers on the relationship between neurology and optometry in the treatment of refractive errors. He has also written a number of books on different problems: dealing with bullies, shedding excess weight, the stock market… He is preparing his next book on risk taking.

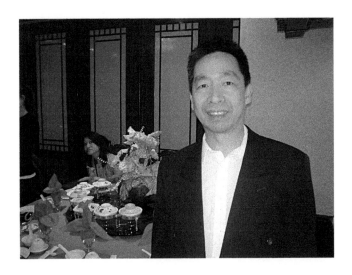

INDEX

1

200 FT. / 61 m

E

20/200

2

100 FT. / 30.5 m

F P

20/100

3

70 FT. / 21.3 m

T O Z

20/70

4

50 FT. / 15.2 m

L P E D

20/50

5

6

7

8

9

10

11

40 FT. | 12.2 m

30 FT. | 9.14 m

25 FT. | 7.62 m

20 FT. | 6.10 m

15 FT. | 4.57 m

13 FT. | 3.96 m

10 FT. | 3.05 m

P E C F D

E D F C Z P

F E L O P Z D

D E F P O T E C

L E F O D P C T

F D P L T C E O

P E Z O L C F T D

20/40

20/30

20/25

20/20

20/15

20/13

20/10

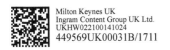